# Body Language

# TRANSITS

## LITERATURE, THOUGHT & CULTURE, 1650–1850

Series editors:
Miriam L. Wallace, University of Illinois Springfield
Mona Narain, Texas Christian University

A landmark series in long-eighteenth-century studies, *Transits* publishes monographs and edited volumes that are timely, transformative in their approach, and global in their engagement with arts, literature, culture, and history. Books in the series have engaged with visual arts, environment, politics, material culture, travel, theater and performance, embodiment, connections between the natural sciences and medical humanities, writing and book history, sexuality, gender, disability, race, and colonialism from Britain and Europe to the Americas, the Far East, the Middle/Near East, Africa, and Oceania. Works that make provocative connections across time, space, geography, or intellectual history, or that develop new modes of critical imagining are particularly welcome.

**Recent titles in the series:**

*Body Language: Medicine and the Eighteenth-Century Comic Novel*
Kathleen Tamayo Alves

*Romantic Beasts: Pervasion, Eccentricity, Exhibition*
Michael Demson and Christopher R. Clason, eds.

*The Art of Retreat: Domestic Romanticisms in the Early United States*
Laurel V. Hankins

*Charles Johnson's "General History of the Pyrates" and Global Commerce*
Noel Chevalier

*Revisiting Richardson*
Rebecca Anne Barr and Bonnie Latimer, eds.

*British Romanticism and Prison Reform*
Jonas Cope

*Prolific Ground: Landscape and British Women's Writing, 1690–1790*
Nicolle Jordan

*Consuming Anxieties: Alcohol, Tobacco, and Trade in British Satire, 1660–1751*
Dayne C. Riley

*The Part and the Whole in Early American Literature, Print Culture, and Art*
Matthew Pethers and Daniel Diez Couch, eds.

For more information about the series, please visit bucknelluniversitypress.org.

# Body Language

## MEDICINE AND THE EIGHTEENTH-CENTURY COMIC NOVEL

KATHLEEN TAMAYO ALVES

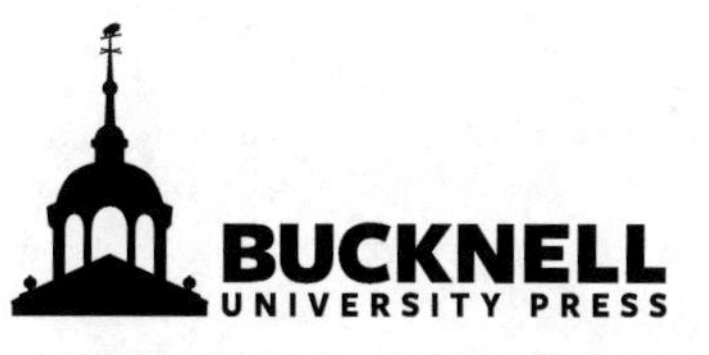


LEWISBURG, PENNSYLVANIA

Library of Congress Cataloging-in-Publication Data

Names: Alves, Kathleen Tamayo, author.
Title: Body language : medicine and the eighteenth-century comic novel / Kathleen Tamayo Alves.
Other titles: Medicine and the eighteenth-century comic novel | Transits (Bucknell University)
Description: Lewisburg, Pennsylvania : Bucknell University Press, 2025. | Series: Transits: literature, thought & culture, 1650–1850 | Includes bibliographical references and index.
Identifiers: LCCN 2025006913 | ISBN 9781684485703 (paperback) | ISBN 9781684485710 (hardcover)
Subjects: LCSH: English fiction—18th century—History and criticism. | English literature—18th century—History and criticism. | Humorous stories, English—18th century—History and criticism. | Medicine in literature. | Women in literature.
Classification: LCC PR448.M42 A48 2025 | DDC 823/.6093561—dc23/eng/20250627
LC record available at https://lccn.loc.gov/2025006913

A British Cataloging-in-Publication record for this book is available from the British Library.



♾ The paper used in this publication meets the requirements of the American National Standard for Information Sciences—Permanence of Paper for Printed Library Materials, ANSI Z39.48-1992.

bucknelluniversitypress.org

Distributed worldwide by Rutgers University Press

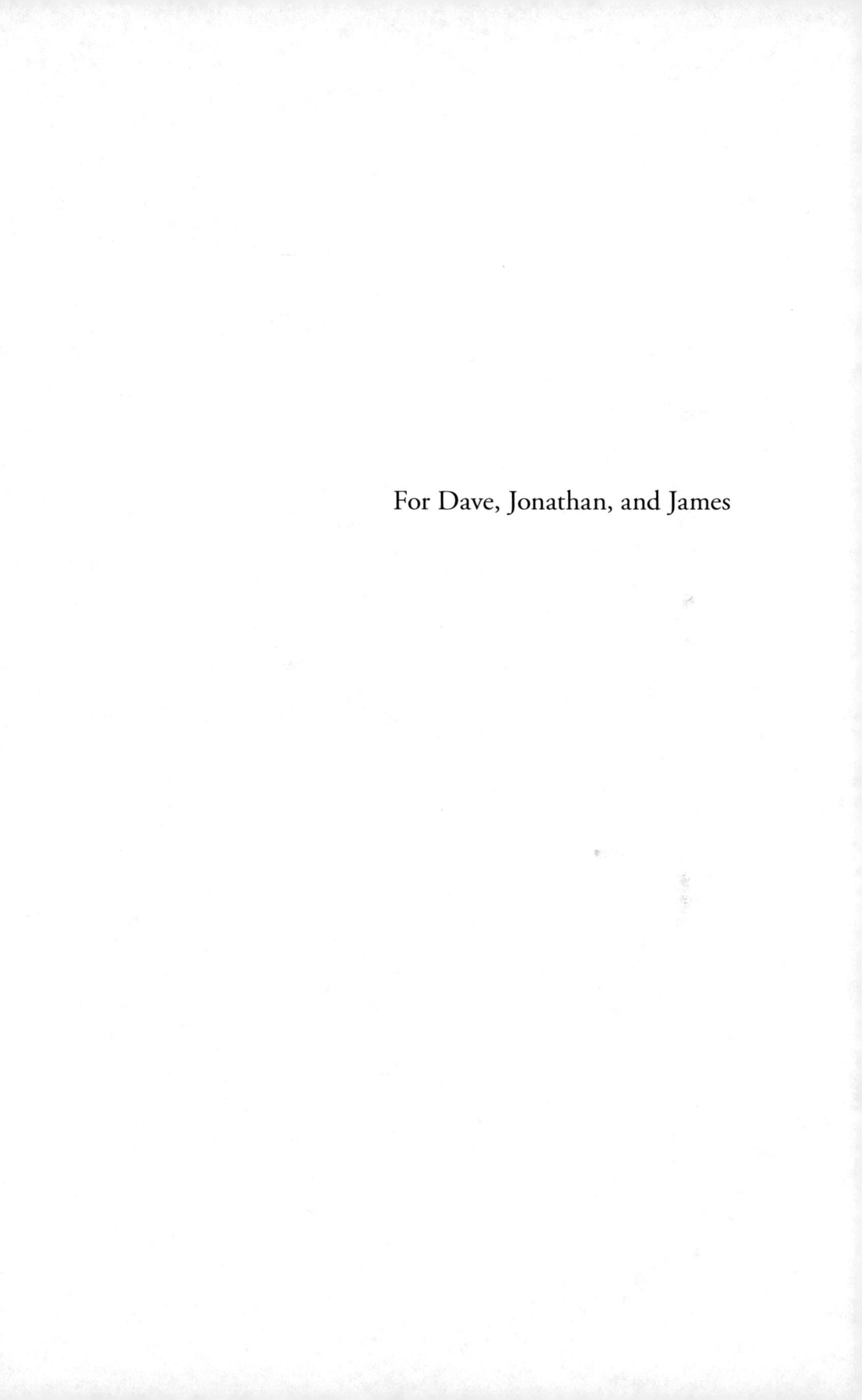

For Dave, Jonathan, and James

# CONTENTS

# Body Language

# INTRODUCTION

## Eighteenth-Century Medicine and Comic Representations of Women

HENRY FIELDING'S *SHAMELA* (1741) FAMOUSLY parodies the "Bundle Scene" in Samuel Richardson's *Pamela* (1740) but with a difference that signifies Shamela's experience. In *Pamela*, the servant heroine rejects the first and second "wicked" bundles as an act of virtuous defiance of her predatory employer, Mr. B. Shamela's bundles include a list of books: didactic works such as Richard Allestree's *Whole Duty of Man* (1658) "with only the Duty to one's Neighbor, torn out"; Methodist George Whitefield's *God's Dealings with Mr. Whitefield* (1740); and coarser material, like Delarivier Manley's *The New Atalantis* (1709/1736), the erotic *Venus in the Cloister; or, The Nun in Her Smock* (1683; trans. 1724), and Lewis Theobald's opera-pantomime *Orpheus and Eurydice* (1739).[1] The wide moral disparity between these works showcases Shamela's symbolic transition from a healthy desexualized childhood to an unhealthy and indecent sexual maturity. The bundles underscore the contrast between Pamela's virtuous naïveté and Shamela's shrewdness, knowing more of society and of men. At fifteen years old, Shamela, perhaps, reached sexual maturity too quickly. Her reading choices (especially *Venus in the Cloister*) may have dangerously excited her imagination and, consequently, her ambition to profit from her sexuality. Pamela's consumption of books was limited to whatever was in her late Lady's library and the Bible; her lack of access to more prurient material preserves her unspoiled nature.

The reading practices of maidservants like Pamela and Shamela reflected a growing concern of the moral influence of the text. The increase of book production, and concomitantly, readers, raised moralist concerns of undisciplined reading habits.[2] One worry was the influence of erotic material on the young woman's imagination, as sexually arousing texts could inflame desires. Medical practitioners agreed that certain books, especially those considered "obscene" like *Venus in the Cloister*, could stimulate a strong sexual appetite and a "coming down" of the menses. During this period, most physicians regarded menstruation as an essentially unclean bodily function, and its onset signaled the transition to a woman's vulnerability to illness for the rest of her life. Therefore, any environmental influence or nonnaturals (like books) that could accelerate this change were considered to be especially pernicious. Furthermore, practitioners even believed that a girl's reading choices could provoke early menarche. The French royal physician Jean Astruc, for instance, asserted that early onset of the menses at ten or eleven years old could be triggered by the "reading of obsene Books, unchast touching, etc. for hereby the Subject becomes a woman as it were before her time."[3] Earlier menstruation meant an earlier sexual awakening that, if not properly controlled or policed, could lead to her destruction. This licentiousness is evident in Shamela's desire for her lover, Parson Williams, with whom she has an illegitimate child. Concurrently, her intemperance extends to her aspirations for upward social mobility through marriage with a country gentleman. Hungry for both, Shamela carries out her campaign of feigned virtue with Booby as she continues to indulge in her sexual relations with Parson Williams: "*O Parson Williams; how little are all the Men in the World compared to thee*" (259). For moralists and physicians, the slippery slope to perdition for prepubescent girls could begin with reading "obsene" books.

This episode in *Shamela*, as in many major novels of humor in the eighteenth century, reveals the reciprocally illuminating connection between literature and medicine. Exploring the cultural interplay between these two realms allows us to consider the links between textual and embodied selves, all set within the context of the historically specific notions of disease and health. Rereading these novels in the context of medical discourse sheds new light on their critical dimensions and has the potential to provide a more comprehensive historical backdrop for their social concerns by highlighting the multifaceted relationships between health, desire, societal order, and gender constructs that were familiar to their readers.

Contributing to the rich body of work in medical humanities in the period, *Body Language* offers an interdisciplinary approach in exploring the intersections of British eighteenth-century comic fiction and medical discourse. Examining medical writings of renowned physicians of the Enlightenment, such as John Freind, Thomas Sydenham, Albrecht von Haller, Robert Whytt, and William Cullen, with novels of humor by Henry Fielding, Tobias Smollett, Laurence Sterne, and Charlotte Lennox, this book explains how medicine shapes comic language in the dramatization of female-specific medical phenomena, such as menstruation, hysteria, nervous disorder, and pregnancy. *Body Language* argues that political and social anxieties broadly centered on women's sexuality, such as their sexual aggression, sexual incontinence, and linguistic intemperance, are problematized within the body (diagnosis and treatment) and expressed through it (symptoms), suggesting that comic works are suspicious of the empirical ethos of scientific objectivity, most especially in the medical recommendation of marriage as a treatment for women's illness.[4]

The comic tradition structures the plots and tropes of these novels: centralizing sex and rebirth, satirizing female affectation, closing with marriage and sexual consummation, and restoring a conservative order in the turbulence of the story's landscape. And yet, through the comic representations of "leaky" female physical, psychological, and emotional embodiment, these novels put into question the efficacy of the institution of marriage as a universal remedy for women's biological and cultural ailments.[5] The pervasive medical notion that women are incapable of bodily self-regulation paradoxically becomes an imperative for policing of women's bodies and highlights the enduring shortcomings of patriarchal systems in maintaining absolute authority. By examining women's sexuality through the medical lens and in the comic mode, I argue that these comic representations offer a counternarrative of women's embodiment, agency, and selfhood, as well as exposing the capacity of the institution of marriage to regulate women's sexuality.

I want to make it clear that the female characters examined in this book and the female bodies examined by eighteenth-century physicians are white. Therefore, it is essential to emphasize that the analyses presented here do not presume to apply universally to women of color, especially when their racial difference justified horrific scientific experimentation, violence, and eugenicist practices.[6] Additionally, it is worth noting that these female characters are assumed to be cisgender, but they are not representative of all people who identified as women. As Susan Lanser has powerfully demonstrated, many in the period lived outside of the "heterosexual dyad" and "transgressed heteronormative rubrics."[7] Michael Warner and Lauren Berlant have identified the eighteenth century as the period in which heteronormativity became central to national identity, with the heterosexual dyad serving as a "tacit but central organizing index of social membership" that produced "utopia[s] of social belonging." Practices that seemed to be irrelevant to sex consolidated a community that governed "in almost every aspect of the forms and arrangements of social life: nationality, the state, and the law; commerce; medicine; and education; as well as in the conventions and affects of narrativity, romance, and other protected spaces and cultures."[8] The medical institution, represented by the writings of medical practitioners referenced in this book, can be seen as reinforcing the consolidation of heterosexual norms by conflating sex and gender with anatomy. The ways these characters perform their gender, whether conforming to or challenging prescribed notions of femininity, underscore the instability of sex and gender, highlighting that neither is self-evident.[9]

While the medical theories explored in this book may differ across chapters, they share a common concern regarding the perceived dangers of excess. Each novel presents a conflict between medical discourse and societal expectations: The former posits that female excess is unmanageable under certain circumstances, while the latter insists that it should always be controlled. The incorporation of medical elements in the comic novel serves as a critique of the irreconcilable clash between medical discourse's portrayal of women's psycho-physiological excess and cultural demands for women to exhibit unwavering sexual virtue. These novelists draw from contemporaneous medical ideas to make the comedy available and immediate for their readers.

## EIGHTEENTH-CENTURY SCIENCE AND GENDER

The eighteenth century is a rich period for examining the naturalization of gender, particularly through the work of male physicians in understanding the female body's mechanisms and its distinctions from the male body. Thomas Laqueur notes that "women's bodies in their corporeal, scientifically accessible concreteness, in the very nature of their bones, nerves, and, most important, reproductive organs came to bear an enormous new weight of cultural meaning in the Enlightenment."[10] Reexamining medicine's and science's role in authenticating gender difference within their historical context becomes crucial for tracing the principles that led to accepted biological truths. Felicity Nussbaum writes, "Sexual difference as historical and cultural configuration allows us to analyze its manifestation in various historical moments and to imagine its reconfiguration because the meaning of a biological 'fact' changes through time. As a result, rather than confusing the metaphors of science with objective truths, biology emerges instead as a powerful representational model that avoids claiming to be an essential reality."[11] Scientific metaphors serve as powerful tools for comprehending the cultural dimensions of gender. Mary Douglas observes, "The human body is always treated as an image of society and . . . there can be no natural way of considering the body that does not involve at the same time a social dimension."[12] As institutions that purportedly depend on empirical methods to determine fact, science and medicine rely on metaphors in their discursive practices, to demystify the mysteries of the human body either to themselves or to their audience. This reliance, at times, draws from preexisting ideas about gender and its available signifiers familiar to the speaking and reading subjects in culture. One consequence of such borrowing is the reinforcement of traditional ideas about gender and sexuality, except it is now bolstered by what could be construed as indisputable biological realities.

Science and medicine were important to Enlightenment explorations of sexuality, as explained by the historian Ludmilla Jordanova.[13] First, natural philosophers and medical writers considered themselves in relation to their experiences in the natural world, such as procreation, sexual behavior, and venereal diseases. Second, the secular, empirical methods of science and medicine occupied an elite epistemological position, departing from dogma and superstition. Empiricism and the experimental method promoted the ideal of objective knowledge derived from theories of observation, the inference of facts from observable nature through the senses or instruments, and the practice of induction, which synthesized answers by the analysis of problems via coherence and completeness of sequence and careful weighing of evidence.[14] In medicine, the emphasis on empiricism and the individual fostered a keener interest in morbid or pathological anatomy and clinical pathology, which relied on quantifiable results.[15] Third, medical writings used sexual metaphors as a vehicle for understanding, for instance, by depicting nature as a woman to be uncovered and penetrated by masculine science. Scientific accounts reiterated deep-rooted stereotypes; from courageous spermatozoon to the timid, passive egg, nature is gendered in scientific narratives.[16] Lynda Birke notes that the emergence of the mechanistic medical worldview accompanied the transformations of gendered metaphors in science. Before 1700, nature was viewed as a nurturing mother of creation, but afterward, the metaphors acquired imperialistic undertones.[17] Christina Larner points out that these metaphors were sexually aggressive, implying that nature's secrets should be torn from her, in a kind of figurative rape.[18] In *The Masculine Birth of Time* (1603), Francis Bacon, hailed as the father of modern science in his era, stressed the necessity of conquering nature through knowledge: "I am come in very truth leading to you Nature with all her children to bind her to your service and make her your slave." Appealing to "true sons of knowledge," Bacon urged male scholars to "penetrate further" to get to her "inner chambers."[19] Nature as female was imagined to be passively ready for such masculine discovery. Evelyn Fox Keller refers to the masculine face of science as a sex act, the central metaphor of scientific discovery.[20]

The associations between women and nature, and between men and culture, often had sexed-based distinctions. The sexual double standard was interpreted as rules that were simply different for men and women; crude biological essentialism became more inflexible and dichotomous due to the influence of scientific and medical discourse by the end of the century. Consequently, science licensed gendered identification, prescribing specific social roles for women based on their physical and mental attributes. Londa Schiebinger observes in her study of late eighteenth-century scientific perspectives on sexuality that anatomists shifted from the outdated humoral framework to a new way of explaining the origins of sexual difference, sexual and gender relations, and sexuality. They began to view sexuality as extending beyond reproductive organs.[21] For instance, the French physician Pierre Roussel criticized fellow practitioners for placing women and men on equal terms, except for differences in sexual organs: "The essence of sex," he argued, "is not confined to a single organ but extends, through more or less perceptible nuances, into every part."[22] Similarly, the German anatomist Jacob Ackermann explained that available definitions of sexual differences fell short since they inadequately described the unique female body. Inspecting every difference between male and female bones, hair, eyes, voices, blood vessels, and brains, Ackermann appealed to doctors to find "the essential sexual difference" from which all others flowed.[23] Schiebinger views this period as a pivotal moment in the history of medicine, for by the 1790s, European anatomists began depicting sexed bodies with specific telos: "physical and intellectual strength for a man, motherhood for the woman."[24] In alignment with these binary categories, internal anatomical differences between men and women became increasingly emphasized, encompassing muscles, bones, and brains.

Examining the portrayal of women in the history of the science, feminist scholars like Jordanova have revealed the mutually reinforcing epistemological connection between science and patriarchy.[25] From this perspective, literary works mirror the period of their production. But literature also serves as a medium for absorbing, relocating, reflecting, incorporating, commenting, and critiquing social norms. Comic works create critical distance from the familiar. *Body Language* aims to complicate this narrative of medical and literary discourse as purely serving or reinforcing patriarchal ideology. By examining the appropriation of medical elements in the comic novel, I suggest that comic works, in particular, reintegrate women's experiences in medical and cultural history, and the incorporation of medical elements in these narratives (deliberately parodic or not) underscores the tensions between medical discourse's opinion of women's psycho-physiological excess and social codes of female sexual virtue.

## THE COMIC NOVEL AND THE GROTESQUE BODY

But what links fictional works and medical texts in the eighteenth century? The answer, broadly stated, is the body. Doctors study the intricacies and mechanisms of the body, while humor finds its expression through bodily experiences. The body, as a tangible object that conveys meaning through reference, is inherently polysemic, accommodating multiple potential interpretations. This polysemy is evident in both the disparate medical understandings of the body and the stylistic variations among comic authors.

As cultural products, both medical and comic texts share multidimensional material space in the public sphere, coevolving and indivisible. Examining their intertextuality opens the seams of reciprocal linguistic traces. Scientific writing, as a distinct discourse with its own specialized language and classification systems, equips itself with conceptual tools that yield a tenable knowledge of the material world. And, as a signifying practice, this language gives meaning to the material object of the body, which shapes sexual subjectivity, translating into concrete cultural practices, like bodily self-regulation. For example, the medical belief that the absence of menstrual flow could transform a female into a male, in both physical features and temperament, aligns with the prevailing moral rhetoric of the period that associated blushing with feminine sexual innocence. Epithets like "the blush of modesty," "the blush of delicacy," and "innocent blush" translated as praise for the virtuous woman. The transient coloring on her cheeks symbolized innocent shame, an attractive quality for potential suitors. Many virtuous heroines, from Richardson's Pamela to Frances Burney's Evelina, blushed as a reflection of their virtuous sensibility. Conversely, comic fiction's satirical take on the cultural discourse of medicine and science exposes the tensions inherent in medical and social subjectivity. This can be seen when Shamela, Fielding's satirical antithesis of Pamela, feigns her blushes on her wedding night to dupe her groom, Mr. Booby, into reading chastity on her face. By the same humoral logic, menopause in women "signalled the reassimilation of the female body to the male (and hence more tractable) body."[26] And yet, the hot flashes these women experienced were viewed as a sign of sexual arousal, the origin of the oversexed older woman cliché. Also, the supposed buildup of black bile that would have been released through regular menstruation was seen as the cause of an older woman's evil thoughts, the root of the "witchy" representations of aging women familiar to us today.[27] The physical symptoms of menopause paradoxically conflated aging women with masculine bodily control and the immoral hypersexuality of the witch. In these ways, scientific discourse has contributed to the constructions and representations of the female body, especially in an age when scientific practice was predominantly the domain of men. In response, the comic novel's portrayals of female bodies cast doubt on the social and scientific legitimacy of these constructions, challenging established norms and beliefs.

Beyond a shared emphasis on the body, generic conventions link scientific writing and comic fiction. They both evolved in tandem, each seeking to exert influence on the structural discourse they inhabited, thereby refining its boundaries and norms. In the early decades of the novel, authors strived for narrative coherence and credibility. This divergence in ethos and style is apparent when comparing, for example, the gritty portrayal of the criminal underworld in Daniel Defoe's *Moll Flanders* (1722) with the domestic drama told through sustained epistolary narrative in Samuel Richardson's *Pamela*. Similarly, the physical sciences endeavored to cultivate a specialized language aimed at systematizing the human body to comprehend its mechanisms. Medicine attempted to tell the story of the body, to apprehend its mysteries, in different and contradictory ways. For instance, physicians battled over the story of the fetus. A bitter controversy over maternal impressions emerged, with imaginationists asserting the indelible impact of the mother's actions and thoughts on the fetus, while anti-imaginationists argued that the fetus lived in a state of neutrality. Lynda Birke aptly concludes, "Biomedical discourse is not, as it is sometimes portrayed, just another master narrative, despite its power. It contains within itself all kinds of contradictory strands and fragmentary positionings. It is a motley collection of narrative, building its tales on a motley collection of human and animal bodies; it is not a unitary story."[28] In other words, the novel and medicine expressed narrative in different and, at times, contradictory ways.

While medical and comic narratives attempted to tell stories about human beings in varying modes, they shared a common ethical purpose. The resilience of medical models can be ascribed to their pursuit of a deeper comprehension of the human experience, encompassing both physical and mental states of well-being and health. In Roy and Dorothy Porter's study of early modern approaches to health, both medical practitioners and laypeople alike recognized illness as an affliction that impacted the entire individual, often attributing specific maladies to idiosyncratic habits.[29] One's constitution determined health, with physical illness often seen as an outward manifestation of moral flaws. The external made the internal visible. The "nonnaturals" were six extrinsic factors to consider in one's health as well. In addition to personal constitutions, one's excesses, deficiencies, or corruptions in excretions, air, exercise, sleeping habits, diet, and passions directly impacted a person's health. Therefore, patients had a significant role in maintaining their health through self-discipline.[30] Though no monolithic medical theory dominated in the period, physicians consistently considered the connections between a person's constitution, behavior, and health in diagnosis and treatment.[31] Patients could manage to stave off symptoms of a disease, even if they were constitutionally predisposed to that disease, as long as they followed a disciplined regimen.[32] Factors like damp air were beyond the patient's control, but other "nonnaturals" were associated with vices, like eating or drinking to excess (gluttony) or sleeping past morning prayers (sloth). And as far as the category of the passions as a "nonnatural," excesses such as lust, rage, or covetousness were believed to contribute to physical illness. For example, the extensive scholarship on venereal disease—illnesses frequently attributed to excessive and potentially fatal carnal appetites—notes the moralizing tone in physicians' writings.[33] In diagnosis, physicians aimed to heal both soul and body.

Medicine's curative properties for the soul provide the most forceful rhetorical parallels with comic fiction.[34] The poet Thomas D'Urfey makes this connection concrete, asserting that "Satyres, just like Medicines, are design'd, / As those the body cure, so these the mind."[35] The poet and dramatist John Dryden, echoing the sentiments of many critics in his time, defended comedy's role in social critique. He argued that wit "causes laughter in those who can judge of men and manners, by the lively representation of their folly and corruption."[36] The defining feature of satire, in Dryden's *Discourse Concerning the Original and Progress of Satire* (1693), is "the scourging of Vice, and Exhortation to Virtue."[37] The objective of comic narrative, according to Alan Ackerman and Magda Romanska, is to produce a transition from "habitual behavior, arbitrary laws, obsession, hypocrisy, and fixed social arrangements to a state that is self-aware, more fluid, honest and creative."[38] The comic mode eases this uncomfortable transition for its audience. In 1709, Lord Shaftesbury articulated the "relief theory" of humor in his "Essay on the Freedom of Wit and Humor," suggesting that laughter releases the tensions built up in the "animal spirits" of the body. Subsequent theories of comedy describe a process in which the audience's anxieties or fears find safe and healthy release in laughter. Comic plots first evoke a feeling of discomfort from the audience that generate tension, leading to a catharsis of laughter, a kind of liberation from the anxiety caused by the initial uneasiness. The philosopher Simon Critchley characterizes this experience as "structured fun," asserting that much of humor possesses a dual nature, simultaneously subversive and conservative. Humor gives its audience a much-needed escape from the routine, mocking people in the higher ranks, then returning to the familiar status quo, even strengthening the hierarchy it temporarily subverted.[39] Given the prevalence of gender hierarchies in British society, the recurring comic motif of the subversive female body, marked by its excess and instability, is unsurprising.

The relationship between the female form and the comic novel is precisely why *Body Language* adopts Mikhail Bakhtin's theory of the grotesque body as its primary theoretical framework. Bakhtin identifies the pudendum and the womb as sites where the grotesque body evacuates itself, emphasizing that this body "is not separated from the rest of the world. It is not a closed, completed unit; it is unfinished, outgrows itself, transgresses its own limits. The stress is laid on those parts of the body that are open to the outside world, . . . the parts through which the body itself goes out to meet the world."[40] The grotesque body closely resembles the female body's porousness and fluidity in its interaction with its environment, although they differ in cultural significance. While the grotesque body, conceptualized within popular festivity, functions as a leveling, antihierarchical, collective political instrument, what Bakhtin calls the "carnivalesque," the woman's bodily difference, characterized as wet and leaky and contrasted with the standards of men's hot and solid bodies, is viewed as inferior by the medical community. Elizabeth Grosz asks whether "the female body has been constructed not only as a lack or absence but with more complexity, as a leaking, uncontrollable, seeping liquid; as formless flow; as viscosity, entrapping, secreting; [as] . . . a formlessness that engulfs all form, a disorder that threatens order." Women may share many of the same anatomical structures as men, but "insofar as they are women, they are represented and live themselves as seepage, liquidity."[41] Birke concludes that "fluidity . . . is seepage out from the body—from the breasts in lactation, from the genitals in sexual desire. To be female is to leak in excess."[42] Consequently, the grotesque female body becomes the deviation to the normalized male body. As Birke points out, "women's bodies are hence other to the supposedly exemplary bodies of male physiological controls, just as a lesbian body is other to an assumed heterosexual one."[43] This construction of otherness is deeply embedded in exclusionary practices within medicine, determining what is considered normal or healthy. Enlightenment medicine is a palimpsest of the Aristotelian idea that woman is an imperfect man, with her inferiority attributed to her body's coolness, while the male body is seen as superior due to its warmth. For Galen, the most influential physician in the ancient world, men's testes were of prime importance in male bodies since they cooked the blood; the female analog, the ovaries, operated in the same way but with less efficiency. As Nancy Tuana figuratively puts it, "Woman remains, so to speak, half baked."[44] As such, the leaky bodies of women in the comic novel play along the edges of disturbing the social peace. Their experiences find brief moments of expression in literary burlesque, which reproduces grotesque depictions of the female body, linguistic diversity, and parody. These celebrations, rather than degradations, highlight the female body's excessive linguistic expression, as envisioned in her "leaky vessel." Ultimately, in adherence to the comic mode, the women that inhabit these bodies often become failures, disregarded, or at best, transformed to conform to the social model of feminine virtue.

In Bakhtinian terms, the grotesque's presence can be understood as a positive but temporary suspension of hierarchy during carnival. Difference can function as an open challenge to the legitimacy of existing structural power relations. This difference, which embodies the spirit of humor and chaos that subverts the assumptions of dominant culture, can be construed as deformity by that system of domination. Medicine is an arm of this system, and its efforts to adjudicate and systematize this difference as a natural fact in the Enlightenment ethos consolidate the regulation of the normative body. In the eighteenth century, as explained by Essaka Joshua, *deformity* was a slippery and debatable category that encompassed any deviation from standards of health and beauty.[45] Joshua demonstrates that deformity involved an observable atypicality in a person's corporeal constitution but did not necessarily imply a physical impairment. And as far as how women were conceptualized under the category of deformity, Helen Deutsch and Felicity Nussbaum observe that women's bodily difference as a cultural trope is sometimes "simply made equivalent to deformity or monstrosity so that women are, by their very nature, deemed to be defective."[46] Furthermore, gender fluidity for men and women (e.g., intersex people, eunuchs, Amazons, fops) became increasingly unnatural and aberrant to the norms of the emerging bourgeois aesthetic. The anonymous author of *Beauty's Triumph, or, the Superiority of the Fair Sex Invariably Proved* (1751) criticizes the distasteful incongruence of women assuming men's gendered roles: "Is it not full as unseemly a sight to behold a *Woman* giving the word of command to her troops, leading them up to combat in battle array, and giving them the signal of onset, as to see a *Man* knotting, knitting, handling a distaff, or embroidering his wife's petticoat? The reason is, that every thing unnatural and out of character is offensive."[47] These clashing concepts—the grotesque and deformity—push against each other in the comic novel in its representations of women. The grotesque challenges systems of domination through ridicule and humor, while the categorization of deformity attempts to reinforce the normative engine of those systems.

## WOMEN ARE A JOKE

The effect of comedy is intuitive. We know a work is comical when it makes us laugh. Defining and theorizing the comic is trickier; the comic mode, in making a mockery of convention and decorum, resists definition. Moreover, explaining what makes something funny can often have the effect of making it unfunny. Nonetheless, theoreticians have forwarded different ideas that contribute to the understanding of the comic and its forms, as a genre, though comic plots and characters since antiquity have persisted to the present day. Sex remains a central feature of comedy, a trope that harks back to Dionysian rites of fertility and phallic processions in ancient Greece. The comic's origin in the playfulness of these ancient rites remains in the structure of the joke, as Mary Douglas has observed.[48] The joke's humor comes from the incongruity between expectation and result. According to the "incongruity theory," developed in the eighteenth century by James Beattie, Francis Hutcheson, and Immanuel Kant, a joke's punch line is incongruous with the setup.[49] Generally, the seven novels examined in this book set up the expectation that women can adhere to (and desire) social codes of sexual virtue, but the punch line, buttressed by medical discourse's belief of women's helplessness against their own psycho-physiological excess, subverts that expectation. Women are the subjects of the joke, but on a broader metatheatric, self-conscious level, the joke is on the absurdities of the male-dominated medical establishment's failures in explaining how women's bodies operate outside of the patriarchal paradigm.

If sex and rebirth are central to comedy, then women's reproductive capacity reconstitutes humor in the eighteenth century, specifically through the intersections of women's bodies as cultural and medical signifiers as virgins, mothers, and widows. In broad terms, women are both sexual and sexualized objects, defined by their physical difference and embodiment. As menstruating virgins, they are primed for conjugal duties through the social and economic contract of marriage, with cisheteronormative reproductive futurity perpetuating oppressive conditions for women. Pregnant women's bodies in *Tristram Shandy* and *Peregrine Pickle* stand as evidence of a reproductive sex act. Fielding's female libertines, such as Lady Booby and Lady Bellaston, desire or participate in nonreproductive sex. All women, to some degree, are potential rape victims. As sexual objects, women in the eighteenth-century comic novel span the spectrum of virgins or whores, and the specter of sexual violence, a recurring element in comedy from antiquity to the Restoration, lurks in the background. In Simon Dickie's extensive analysis of the rape joke in the eighteenth century, he illustrates how sexual violence functioned as a flexible metaphor and plot device. The difference in the comic plot is the narrative consequences of rape: the heroine's escape, either on her own or with the help of her hero, and the humbling of the heroine's pride for a suitable marriage.[50] Lennox's *The Female Quixote* can then be characterized as one long rape joke, with

Arabella's unrelenting fears of male sexual predation. *The Female Quixote*'s conclusion with Arabella's marriage to Glanville allows the novel to remain within the realm of comedy. Even *Tristram Shandy*'s final joke of Obadiah's wife being impregnated by Walt's bull, who "might have done for Europa herself in purer times," alludes to a rape from mythology.[51]

Marriage and sexual consummation, since the Greek New Comedy, commonly close the standard comic plot, signaling a new social compact between lovers and the transition from bondage to freedom.[52] In contrast to the tragic ending, in which the hero dies a lonely death that severs him from his community, the comic ending signifies a lasting bond between lovers and the promise of renewal through the birth of offspring, the inevitable product of heterosexual sex.[53] The social ritual of marriage moves beyond a vow between lovers; it denotes a public commitment to the continuity and survival of the community as a whole. Although the world of the comic may be temporarily disrupted, the wedding finale could be interpreted as a reaffirmation of the existing patriarchal order. *Humphry Clinker*, *Joseph Andrews*, *Tom Jones*, *Peregrine Pickle*, and *The Female Quixote* all conclude with couplings (*Tristram Shandy* is the outlier in the group, though the husband's anxiety over healthy issue drives much of the novel). Often, the road to the novel's end is riddled with obstacles created by women in excess. These women need to be overcome, humbled, or punished to maintain the equilibrium of the social contract. The medical framing of women's bodies as both naturally and unnaturally leaky contributes to the common prescription of marriage and motherhood as the cure. And yet, pleasure-seeking widows, like Lady Booby and Lady Bellaston, and monstrous mothers, like Sally Pickle, stand as failures of this prescribed cure. Even as these novels adhere to the comic structure of the wedding or marriage as the happy ending, the novels themselves critique the oppressive ideology of marriage for women. So, then, whose happy ending is it?

The excesses of women are represented for comic effect in wordplay, raillery, burlesque, or parody, but they also serve as subjects of comic irony, women whose pretentions need to be deflated to unblock the happiness of other, more deserving characters for the happy ending. The structural plots of these novels align more closely with the idealism of the romance. Northrop Frye describes the spectrum of comic structures with pure satire on one end and romance on the other. For Frye, romance is propelled by love as both a force and a goal, not only where lovers are reunited but also where long-lost siblings and parents find reconciliation. Romantic idealism, in this context, is not lofty but domestic, with harmony established within marriage and the home. This harmony also entails an economic restoration, with the material futures of characters secured.[54] To reach this happy ending, the agents who are impeding the happiness of the deserving need to be exposed and at times punished. Thus, these novels have implicit or explicit satirical aims to restore social and domestic order. For instance, Shamela's affectation is a dangerous femininity that threatens class hierarchy and the possible contamination of genteel family lineage with the blood of the lowborn, while Winifred Jenkins's affectation is viewed as positive and charming, posing no harm to the family bloodline by marrying a fellow servant. Mrs. Trunnion, Sally Pickle, and Elizabeth Shandy attempt to assert authority over their pregnant bodies but are undermined, either by themselves or by male authority figures who claim to know more about their bodies than they do. Lady Booby and Lady Bellaston's oversexed, jealous characters cause trouble for the hero and conventionally virtuous heroine. Arabella's heightened sense of pride, stemming from her romantic education, hinders her from achieving domestic felicity with her cousin. Thus, there is very little room for unruly, leaky women in the cultural imagination of domestic happiness.

So, are the satirical purposes of these novels progressive or conservative? It remains unclear, and this ideological ambiguity has been the focal point of much debate on the comic.[55] Lauren Berlant and Sianne Ngai observe, "There is something internal to comedy—maybe its capacity to hold together a greater variety of manifestly clashing or ambiguous affects—that makes its boundaries so uniquely ambiguous."[56] Not only does comedy, as Berlant and Ngai suggest, briefly alleviate anxiety, but "its action just as likely produces anxiety: risking transgression, flirting with displeasure, or just confusing things in a way that both intensifies and impedes the pleasure."[57] For Bakhtin, the novel's capacity to absorb and transform other modes and representations makes it difficult to pin down a single, monolithic teleology, and the range of intersubjective forms we encounter in humor reminds us of their existence even as we laugh at them. And if eighteenth-century critics insist that comedy should only poke fun at corrigible imperfection, women's leakiness should not be funny, as it is beyond their control. However, that leakiness can serve as a target of comic ridicule if the leaky woman aspires to assume a subjectivity beyond her prescribed social role. In this sense, the satire is conservative, as it defends the ethical standards and social decorum of its time. And yet, perhaps more subtly, these novels also take up the failures of medical discourse in explaining how women's bodies function and how the institution of marriage continues to fail women. The radical implication demystifies marriage as a life stage when women are freed from bondage (e.g., their father's thumb or economic precarity) and sickness (e.g., hysteria or greensickness from virginity). In an age when medical practice becomes increasingly professionalized and male dominated, especially in fields like obstetrics that were previously dominated by women, scientific reasoning impedes, rather than advances, women's parity within the gender dynamics of power.

This book is interested in the literary and medical articulations of the female body as a cultural signifier and the stories this body tells. I examine the cultural codes embedded in models of human physiology in which the body operates as a site of the struggle between meaning and truth in the realm of science. Social constructionism often promotes false dualities of nature and culture, body and mind, even as it attempts to disavow them. Meaning to move beyond these polarities, some critics have promoted more phenomenological approaches to understanding the body as a lived experience. For Grosz, the body is not just a biological entity but also simultaneously a signifier and a signified; the body becomes "a body as social and discursive object, a body bound up in the order of desire, signification, and power."[58] These significations operate within the internal constitution of the body or theories of how biological systems work and the external relationships of the female body within cultural perspectives of moral value. Social judgments advance particular narratives that establish rules of reference from which individuals are constituted as cultural subjects. For instance, the absence of menstrual flow in the male body was seen as proof of robust health and efficiency, with the abnormality specific to the female body in contrast.[59] Thus, medical practitioners argued that women needed to regulate their behavior since their bodies were more precariously balanced than those of males. This policing of bodily excess translated into linguistic regulation, exemplified in the linguistic reserve of Fielding's heroines, such as Sophia Western in *Tom Jones*, identifying them as desirable, virtuous women characters. The way in which the female body has been imagined by medical science exhibits the paradox of agency and discipline. While medicine has been deeply implicated in the disciplining and surveillance of modern society, as Michel Foucault has explained in his corpus, from *Madness and Civilization* (1961) to *The History of Sexuality* (1978), the active and interventionist body also possesses the potential for generative or productive acts alongside self-restraint. Social regulation processes, such as linguistic parameters, are constitutive of self-fashioning of conduct and ethical competency. The comic novel's representations of the female's "grotesque" body, I believe, encapsulate the tensions arising from this paradox of female agency and discipline.

## OVERVIEW OF THE BOOK

This book is structured thematically, with each chapter focusing on a specific branch of medicine that theorizes the female body's pathologies rooted in its imagined excess. I address medical ideas of the male body in juxtaposition to the female body, underlining the binary oppositions created in science and its contributions to the greater patriarchal discourses in culture that reinforce and naturalize female inferiority. To comprehensively examine the interconnected components of both the novel and medical discourse as integral parts of a dynamic system, I juxtapose literary texts with physicians' writings. Some sections of this study rely more heavily on the work of particular physicians (e.g., chapters 1 and 4), while other sections cast a wider net, encompassing a variety of medical texts. This study does not aspire to be exhaustive; instead, it delves into areas of medicine that investigate the inner and outer workings of the female body and novels of humor that most vividly articulate these medical narratives. The organization of this book is not strictly chronological, primarily because the contentious nature of medical discourse throughout modern history defies a linear narrative structure, with physicians building on or utterly disavowing past ideas and practices.

Chapter 1 discusses how the malapropistic writings of maidservants in *Humphrey Clinker* (1771) and *Shamela* articulate discursive elements of what Bryan Turner calls a "somatic society," one in which major political and personal concerns are both problematized within the body and expressed through it.[60] Linking menstruation theory advanced by John Freind in *Emmenologia* and the maidservant's linguistic excess in Fielding's *Shamela* and Smollett's *Humphry Clinker*, I consider comic fiction's parody of scientific discourse as an expression of female subjectivity regulated by medicalization. While Shamela and Winifred Jenkins's writings, which I characterize as grotesque representations of literacy, are imbued with physical obscenity that draws attention to their sexuality, they also express the novel's engagement with the leaky female underclass body as envisioned in iatromechanical menstruation theory and humor. Chapter 2 examines medical histories of hysteria alongside the hysteric expressions of Fielding's libertine women, Lady Booby in *Joseph Andrews* and Lady Bellaston in *Tom Jones*. While they are cast as the lovesick villains in the novels, these women's emotional struggles are articulated through their speech and writing shaped by amatory language, rendering them as both comic and sympathetic subjects. This chapter questions medical discourse's imposition of a particular vision of women's emotional embodiment in their experience and expressions of desire, the ways in which problematic female sexuality in the guise of libertine excess demonstrates that Enlightenment self-determination is reserved only for men, as women's bodily experiences always operated within cultural norms. Chapter 3 explores the culture of pregnancy and women's ways of knowing in Laurence Sterne's *Tristram Shandy* (1759) and Smollett's *Peregrine Pickle* (1751). Both novels engage with several debates concerning the art of obstetrics—parental attribution, midwifery, sham practitioners—that essentially discredit women's epistemological authority over their own bodies. Childbirth and pregnancy had long been fields dominated by women practitioners, and the increasingly male-dominated field of obstetrics worked to reinforce gender domination in medicine and culture. Finally, chapter 4 is interested in the tensions regarding the culture of sensibility, reading, and women's bodies in Lennox's *The Female Quixote* (1752). Building on chapter 2's discussions on hysteria, I look to the early vitalists of the period, primarily the Scottish physician Robert Whytt, and how this early form of neurology explains the gap between Arabella's intelligence and presumed insanity shaped by her reading of French romances. Arabella's genuine emotional responses to potential male violence, deployed as the main source of humor in the novel, emphasize an uncomfortable (and inconvenient) truth about the sentimental conceptualization of the family, courtship, and marriage.

The female characters discussed in this book largely fall within the spectrum of negative femininity, regarded as charming in their social faux pas, as seen with Smollett's Winifred Jenkins, or as dangerous in their villainous machinations, as exemplified by Fielding's Lady Bellaston. My intention is to open the conversation between readers and scholars, to reexamine these women as whole, autonomous human beings who have been subjected to unattainable standards of decorum and, in my greater argument, standards of health. Both the comic novel and medical writing are textual forms that endeavor to express the lived experiences of human beings. Through these spaces, I aim to uncover the cracks and tensions at the edges, to discover the ideological underbelly of eighteenth-century medical discourse.

Humor is a multifaceted force, simultaneously subversive and conservative, evoking discomfort from its audience that generates tension, then a cathartic liberation from the anxiety caused by this discomfort, ultimately returning to the status quo. In this context, I contend that masculine anxiety propels the literary and medical representations of women's bodies, driven by fear of their excess and liquidity, which entire discursive systems have been constructed to conquer. The comic mode provides a platform to parody these discursive systems and laughs at them, however briefly.

# 1

# LEAKY WRITINGS AND LEAKY BODIES IN HENRY FIELDING'S *SHAMELA* (1741) AND TOBIAS SMOLLETT'S *HUMPHRY CLINKER* (1771)

ON OCTOBER 20, 1702, DR. JOHN FREIND, not yet a fellow of the Royal College of Physicians or attending physician to Queen Caroline, begins treatment for a twenty-four-year-old laundry maid "of sanguine habit" for symptoms resulting from the extended suppression of her menses. Freind did not administer a cure for her flux's yearlong absence, noting that this was of no "remarkable detriment to her Health." He attributed her condition to her underclass constitution, "having been much accustomed to Labour and Exercise." When she began experiencing symptoms such as "heaviness and weakness of Body, Indigestion, a Pain in almost all her Limbs, a Cough, Dyspnaea [labored breathing], a Paleness," swelling of the legs, and, most seriously, the appearance of a tumor, Freind administered the three treatments for such cases: "1. To restore a good Digestion in the Stomach. 2. To increase the Impulse of the Blood. 3. To relax the uterine Vessels."[1] By November 11, all symptoms of her distemper had disappeared. He included this case among others in *Emmenologia* (1703), an influential medical text on menstruation theory based on Newtonian mechanical principles.

Freind was one of many elite medical practitioners, including John Clarke, Thomas Denman, John Haighton, Alexander Hamilton, James Hamilton, John Harvie, William Hunter, John Leake, William Lowder, Colin Mackenzie, John Maubray, William Osborne, William Saunders, William Smellie, and Thomas Young, who contributed to the field of gynecology or obstetrics. The period witnessed a growing interest among general-practice physicians in the realm of midwifery and menstruation theory. These practitioners drew from different models to develop new and more comprehensive explanations regarding the menses that both departed from and shared with many of their predecessors' theories. For example, as an iatromechanist, Freind believed that the body obeyed the same laws of physics as celestial bodies. However, he also frequently cited Hippocrates, who associated disease with environmental factors, in *Emmenologia* as the authority on menstruation mechanics. Despite the eagerness of many medical authorities to explain the causes of menstruation, no single theory dominated medical practice.

The three major theories—response to lunar forces, fermentation of the blood, and plethora—rarely associated menstruation with reproduction. Instead, catamenia was often described in terms of the inherent vulnerabilities of the female body. The absence of menstrual flow in the male body was seen as evidence of its robust health and effectiveness, emphasizing the specific difference in the female body.

Practitioners have maintained that women should regulate their behavior since their bodies were more precariously balanced than those of males. Ultimately, menstruation theory reinforced the female body's ideological marking as a confounding and delicate object. As demonstrated in Freind's case, different kinds of female bodies, like those from the laboring class, experienced their menstrual cycles differently based on constitution and climate, but their "leakiness" continued to mark their bodies as inherently inefficient.

As a leaky site, the pudendum discharges liquid matter and, hence, is one of the few sites of evacuation that Bakhtin aligns with the grotesque body.[2] While the grotesque body shares similarities with the model of the humoral body in its porousness and fluidity with the environment, the two differ in cultural meaning. The grotesque body, conceptualized within popular festivity, functions as a leveling, antihierarchical, collective political instrument of the carnivalesque. On the other hand, the humoral body in the scientific model accentuates women's difference and physical inferiority *because* they menstruate. The comic novel replicates these social tensions and contradictions between the intellectual elite, or the scientific community, and the popular in its parodic representations of underclass women's linguistic styles. Through the literary burlesque, comic writers such as Henry Fielding and Tobias Smollett reproduce grotesque representations of the female body, linguistic diversity, and taste for parody that reclaim underclass feminine selfhood through excessive linguistic expression as imagined in women's "leaky vessel."

This chapter discusses how female underclass writing articulates discursive elements of what Bryan Turner calls a "somatic society," one in which "major political and personal problems are both problematized within the body and expressed through it."[3] The political and personal concerns, broadly speaking, reside within the uncontrollable flows of the woman's body, which also represented her inability to control herself. These problems manifested in fears of sexual, social, and moral contamination from the underclass woman's inability to exercise self-restraint. Linking menstruation theory in the period advanced by Freind in *Emmenologia* and the maidservant's linguistic excess in Henry Fielding's *Shamela* (1741) and Tobias Smollett's *Humphry Clinker* (1771), I consider comic fiction's parody of scientific discourse as an expression of female subjectivity regulated by medicalization. While Shamela's and Winifred Jenkins's writing, which I characterize as grotesque representations of literacy, is imbued with physical obscenity that draws attention to their sexuality, it expresses the novel's engagement with the leaky female underclass body imagined in iatromechanical menstruation theory and humor. Similar to the ways Jared S. Richman views the materiality of speech in print as rendering disabled bodies visible, the comic novel's appropriation of the female underclass through the epistolary form focuses the materiality of speech through this specific body.[4] Comic language's liberating effects articulate the disruptive and expanding potential of servant writing, a revolutionizing influence on the linguistic structures of the novel.

Although all bodies flowed through sweat and blood, ideological markings gradually enclosed the flowing humoral body in the period. With menstruation, female bodily function indicated what Gail Kern Paster calls "uncontrol," therefore becoming a function of gender.[5] This attribution was further naturalized through the complex classification of bodily fluids in Galenic humoralism in theory and practice. This dimorphism complicates Thomas Laqueur's conclusions on the emergence of the two-sex model of the body in the eighteenth century. The previous framework adhered to the Galenic one-sex, male-centric, hierarchical model, which conceptualized male and female bodies in the same way: Women's bodies were imagined to be analogous, inverted versions of men's bodies, and the idea of sex depended on illustrative degrees of perfection, not biological difference.[6] Laqueur's argument possesses a wide currency among scholars despite its critics. The one-sex model's linear trajectory has been scrutinized for its failure to account for the complexities of seventeenth-century medicine, notably by Jonathan Sawday, Janet Adelman, Gianna Pomata, and Helen King.[7] The distinct difference in treatment based on a woman's menstrual functions suggests that male and female bodies were imagined differently. It is within this space of difference that the comic mode plays with the ideological energies shaping cultural and medical narratives around particular bodies. In the case of the underclass female body, her language, framed within the comic model, rewrites the traditional narratives that have negatively represented her as intemperate in body and speech. Her linguistic intemperance, like menstruation, becomes an expression of abundance and possibility, asserting a life and selfhood outside her employer's authority.

## *SHAMELA*

*Shamela* marks Fielding's initial foray into the realm of fiction. Written in a month and initially published anonymously after the release of Samuel Richardson's *Pamela*, *Shamela* satirizes Pamela's hyperbolic moralizing, Richardson's "puffs" in *Pamela*'s prefatory material and the absurdity of the heroine's "writing to the moment," the self-engrossed style of the poet laureate Colley Cibber, and Methodist enthusiasm. Martin Battestin credits Fielding with bringing the "art of parody to near perfection"; *Shamela*'s comic abridgment closely imitates the form and substance of *Pamela* with impressive fidelity.[8] Thomas Lockwood calls *Shamela* "the purest parody Fielding ever wrote, and for that matter one of the purest parodies to be found anywhere on the shelf of the period literature."[9] *Shamela* adheres to the fundamental structure of Richardson's plot but reverses its central premise, turning *Pamela*'s predatory Mr. B into the pliable Squire Booby, and Richardson's pious paragon into the calculating and sexually vigorous Shamela. And in this parody, *Shamela* taps into cultural anxieties surrounding excessive underclass sexuality and burgeoning servant literacy, all within the context of the medical scrutiny of underclass bodies. Through her letters, Shamela rewrites a distinctly assertive femininity that undermines the prevailing social and medical notions that underclass women do not conform to the model of a real woman.

In Shamela's capacity to perform the genteel, bourgeois female body for her own mercenary ends, her body figures as grotesque and antihierarchical. She challenges bourgeois notions of feminine virtue—the female ideal represented by Pamela—as inauthentic, unsustainable, and performative.[10] Writing on eighteenth-century domestic fiction and the making of the modern subject, Nancy Armstrong locates *Pamela*'s importance in the cultural shift from the social contract to the sexual contract that requires women to "relinquish political control to the male in order to acquire exclusive authority over domestic life, emotions, taste, and morality."[11] In these narratives, the woman is rewarded with economic security in exchange for her submission to her husband. For Armstrong, this implies that an autonomous self outside of the sexual contract exists: "If a servant girl could claim possession of herself as her own first property, then virtually any individual must similarly have a self to withhold or give in a modern form of exchange with the state."[12] In Fielding's reframing of *Pamela*, Shamela, in her linguistic intemperance, relinquishes no political control to her husband through her performance of leisure-class delicacy and Christian chastity before and after her marriage to Squire Booby. Her lack of restraint, akin to a woman's inability to control her menses, flows out of her in epistolary speech that asserts an individuality and a membership with the servant community independent of her employer and, later, her husband.

### *Servant Disembodiment and Speech*

There is a double imperative to regulate Shamela's underclass and female body to maintain the sex and class system of governance and domination. Employers feared the potential sexual, social, and moral contamination from the maidservant's excess, especially given her proximity within the household. The female body's social construction as lacking the capacity for self-control is closely tied to prevailing medical notions regarding menstruation. One disciplinary mechanism used to control this potentially contaminating "seepage" is to empty out the maidservant from any sense of selfhood and community, a strategy Shamela actively resists.

Unlike Pamela, Shamela rejects the demand for disembodiment imposed on servants. This rejection is all the more significant in a period when employers actively sought to strip servants of any marker of individuality.[13] And, according to Cissie Fairchilds, this obliteration or scrutiny of personal identity was especially prevalent among maids who were in closer proximity to their mistresses, as was the case with Pamela.[14] Servants were emptied out of their personal histories, their acquaintances, and even their names, which served as markers of a selfhood independent from their employers. In this manner, the servant's presence within the household primarily existed to reaffirm the centrality of the employer's power and identity.

Though employers sought to disembody servants from their individual histories, servant speech became a means of asserting their selfhood beyond the confines of the employer-servant relationship. Georg Lukács noted that, traditionally, the figure of the servant in the early comic novel had no existence outside of servitude and operated only as an ancillary for their employers.[15] However, Bruce Robbins offers a revisionist counterpolitics of the servant in literary and cultural history, emphasizing the individuality of the servant expressed through dialogue and narration. In this way, alternate worlds or futures are imagined through the humor of servant speech. When servants express impertinence, there is a temporary suspension of the employer's authority to enforce deferential silence. In Booby and Shamela's first spirited verbal exchange, he interrupts her reading of *A Short Account of God's Dealings with the Reverend Mr. George Whitefield* (1740) and asks, "What Book is that, I warrant you Rochester's Poems." Her reply ("No, forsooth") unleashes a litany of insults: "Why how now Saucy Chops, Boldface." "Mighty pretty words, says I, pert again." "You are a d—d, impudent, stinking, cursed, confounded Jade, and I have a great Mind to kick your A—." "You, kiss—says I" (317). Shamela's impertinent responses cast her in the higher role of commentator (doubling in authority as the letter writer in the narrative) on Booby's language as a gentleman and her employer. As Robbins has observed,

> Servant speech derives a peculiar power from its multidirectionality. If dialogue is imagined primarily as verbal exchange—whether as the moral ideal of mutual responsiveness or the political reflection of conflicting interests and ideologies—then the tendency of the servant voice is to project itself out of dialogue and into monologue—into a monologue, however, that is at once audience oriented and self-assertive. Nothing could be further from solipsism. The themes, the specific verbal resources, and the general aesthetic authority for the servant's self-assertion derive from the audience, a second and sovereign master. Where masters and servants confront each other, the audience introduces a crucial third term, one that is not reflected in the mirror of mimesis. Thus it might be more accurate to think of dialogue according to a secondary definition, that is, the literary genre of dialogue, in which exchange between speakers is a more

> or less transparent device subordinated to the overriding aim of rhetorical impact.[16]

By shifting the reader's attention to Booby's own rude language, Shamela turns the discourse from a conversation between herself and her employer (who himself fails to adhere to the rhetorical practices of his class and gender) to a wider audience that identifies with the servant's point of view. As I have previously discussed in this book's introduction, Booby expects Shamela to be reading lascivious material (and, admittedly, she does own a copy of *Venus in the Cloister*). Her repudiation of reading preferences subverts the classist assumptions often attributed to servant maids in general, that they were more likely to read smut than sermons. Moreover, calling his insults "mighty pretty words" opens a second rhetorical dimension that moves beyond the present moment of servant impertinence to a linguistic space energized by radical social dissatisfaction. Shamela's responses not only undermine Booby's attempt to demean, objectify, and dehumanize her but also point to the thin, and perhaps false, ideology behind the male gentility and authority that he represents. In her sassy retorts, Shamela refuses to willfully relinquish a selfhood that her employers demand from her, thereby refusing to submit to their absolute authority.

### *(In)Authentic Servant Writing*

Much like how menstruation signified fertility and future possibilities through its abundance and excess, Shamela's letters envision a new world, a revolution quietly orchestrated in servant spaces against predatory wealthy men. What is exceptional about this kind of rebellion is that it tries to game the same system that has historically oppressed women on the basis of the gender ideologies of virtue and female fragility. After refusing Booby's offer to become his mistress, Shamela reveals her ultimate ambition to her mother, Henrietta Andrews: "I thought once of making a little Fortune by my Person. I now intend to make a great one by my Vartue" (329–330). These words were never penned by Pamela, but Pamela's power of virtuous refusal, in the face of material profit, became fodder for satire; many of Richardson's critics found the idea of a maidservant who considered her chastity as a commodity as preposterous.[17] *Shamela*, on the other hand, presents the "true" letters of the real Pamela, a "sham" who feigns chastity, or "vartue," in her own words: "I value my Vartue more than I do any thing my Master can give me," she writes to Henrietta (325).

At first glance, the bastardization of "virtue" to "vartue" might appear to render the maidservant's voice more authentic to her class (like how Smollett shapes Winifred Jenkins's linguistic character through phonetic spelling). Anti-Pamelist readers noted the liberal license Richardson took with Pamela's diction and style. Fielding exaggerates this distinction in *Shamela* by ridiculing Richardson's narrative through linguistically playful and more precise substitutions, such as transforming Pamela's "virtue" to Shamela's explicitly economically driven "vartue."[18] By using orthography as a device for criticism, Catherine Ingrassia observes, Fielding asserts a "distinctive knowingly optical voice that punctures the absurdities of Richardson's fiction and a culture that embraced it so fully."[19] To be sure, Fielding's parodic imitation of Richardson's epistolary style, language, characters, and situations and the moral of *Pamela* exposes its preposterousness.[20] Shamela's performative "vartue" misleads and ultimately ensnares the unsuspecting Booby, all while she is engaging in an intensely carnal affair with Parson Williams. As Michael McKeon observes, this can be seen as a form of Machiavellian *virtù*, a "corrupted term that embodies its own contradictory negation."[21] Additionally, if we consider servant wordplay, as Robbins proposes, as a "kind of pastoral," with its "intermittent reach outside the semantic field of the drama, responding to the extra-dramatic presence and interests of the audience . . . like a brief subliminal glimpse of another society," I offer another reading of "vartue" in place of its common interpretation as a signifier of moral and linguistic corruption.[22] Rather, the servant wordplay of "vartue" extends beyond the novel's landscape, encouraging the book's audience to imagine a possible society in which underclass women like Shamela find empowerment as a community, even as employers actively sought to deindividualize and defeminize them by stripping from them kinship relations. Initially, Shamela sought to make "a little Fortune" by her "Person," perhaps through a sexual contract with Booby. Encouraged by Mrs. Jewkes, Booby's housekeeper, who anticipates that Shamela will "shortly be Mistress of the Family" (329), the maidservant's ambitions rose, to make a "great one" by her "Vartue." Unlike Pamela, Shamela radically reclaims underclass femininity that does not relinquish the self in marriage. Shamela's keenly conscious linguistic and bodily performance of virtuous femininity protects her spirited autonomy, asserting a self that does not bend to her employer's or her husband's will, a self that is all her own.

## The Defeminization of Maidservants

Shamela correctly delineates the different values between a maidservant's and a gentlewoman's body. Each body has a different price, with one worthier than the other for a lifetime of comfort and leisure that comes with marriage. Servants, while frequently hypersexualized in the cultural imagination, are also frequently masculinized and not seen as "real women."[23] This classist perspective finds support from medical practitioners, who often described laboring women with irregular menstrual cycles or amenorrhea (absence of menses) as exhibiting masculine characteristics in behavior, with some theorists going as far as claiming that these menstrual disorders could transform women into intersex beings. Freind claims, "That those Women in whom the Menses have been found wanting, were Viragos, of a very hot Constitution; who since they approach near to the masculine

Robustness, and are very much accustomed to Labour, easily digest all their Aliment, and discharge it thro' the Pores."[24] Like men, laboring women do not discharge bodily fluids through menstruation but through sweat. John Leake wrote in his two-volume *Chronic Diseases Peculiar to Women* (1781) that women who did not menstruate were "commonly robust, and possessed the temperament and disposition of men; barren and bold, they are endowed with masculine feelings, and little susceptible of that tender partiality which mutually influences the two sexes, and endears them to each other; which softens and harmonises the passions of the one, and renders the other irresistibly pleasing."[25]

While physicians like Freind pronounced their knowledge of the female body via empirical observation, their approaches resulted in a distorted view of women's bodies. In Alexandra Lorde's contribution on the period's theories of menstruation, she shows how physicians' population samples, limited to charity hospitals with poor and undernourished women, skewed their findings. Physicians failed to connect gestation and menstruation in this sample since these women continued to become pregnant even when there were long gaps in their cycles, especially in the winter months, when food was scarce.[26] Additionally, the physician-controlled narrative of underclass bodies presumed that women who suffered from amenorrhea developed masculine temperament, with increased aggression and callousness.[27] Freind supposes that "after a long suppression of the Menses, the Body at length so much resembled a man's, as that they became very hairy and bearded."[28] Although the menses were not completely attributed as a female function until toward the end of the century, a healthy, consistent menstrual cycle was a defining feature of womanhood in Freind's estimation.[29] Therefore, the absence of "normal" menstrual function masculinized underclass women with amenorrhea without considering their material realities. Meanwhile, medical theories of chlorosis, or "greensickness," were linked with affluent lifestyles, diagnosing the disease as one of "refinement," even though records show that most of the women who experienced this disorder were from the underclass.[30]

The difference in diagnosis and treatment of women from different social groups demonstrates the reification of class-coded femininity as an exclusionary medical practice. In particular, the attribution of hirsuteness with amenorrhea implies the fluidity of gender representation of underclass women and, perhaps, the latent possibility of transgressive lesbian desire—the kind of which we see represented in Daniel Defoe's Amy in *Roxana* and Mrs. Jewkes in *Pamela*. Ula Klein has written of the significance of the beard's representation in cross-dressing women narratives: "The beard, in its many meanings and its cultural attachment to erotic discourses—masculinity, homosexual hiding, sexual virility, female pubic hair, and rampant female sexuality—emerges as a term whose meaning may vacillate, yet its historically constructed genealogy indicates its persistence."[31] While beards on men, according to Jacques-Antoine Dulaure in *Pogonologia* (1786), are symbols of "[men's] sovereignty," bearded women are "one of those extraordinary deviations with which nature presents us every day."[32] Masculine markers of physicality and personality attributed to underclass women moved them farther away from the feminine end of the gender spectrum, representing them as grotesque and dangerous versions of women.[33] This is all to say that medical readings of sexed bodies carried confirmation bias of existing notions of gender and class codes. The ability to menstruate is a significant marker of a woman in relation to a man. In Freind's and Leake's logic, men are men because they do not menstruate; therefore, women who menstruate irregularly or not at all are considered more physically and emotionally proximate to men than to women. Not only do Pamela's letters and journals enact her virtue (which insist on an inherent, genuine, and nonperformative dimension), but they also attempt to undermine the notion that, as a servant, she is not a woman in the first place.

## *Performing (In)Authentic Femininity*

The equivocal notion of gender and class as performance is perhaps why Fielding's farcical rendering of Shamela's experience underscores her deliberate performance of virtue in her interactions with Booby. Thomas Lockwood noted that Shamela's characterization drew from Fielding's theatrical experience, particularly the sassy soubrettes and other leading ladies in the plays he specifically wrote for the famous comedienne Catherine Clive.[34] Shamela's fake fainting fits, a comic reversal of the attempted rape scene in *Pamela*, satirize both Richardson's style of Pamela's "writing to the moment" and her fragile sensibility: "I counterfeit a swoon. . . . O what a Difficulty it is to keep one's Countenance, when a violent Laugh desires to burst forth" (318). Shamela's seeming to be what she is not echoes the concern of writers like Jonathan Swift, Joseph Addison, and Richard Steele that women's bodies, adorned with ornamentation, expose them of artifice. If women, as Pope supposes in his *Epistle to a Lady* (1735), "have no Characters at all," then there is nothing to discover under all their deceit.[35] These sentiments betray a masculine anxiety of women's control over their own bodies and appearance. If the discourse of medicine reinforces men's overall bodily superiority, grounded in their ability to maintain bodily self-possession, then women, as "leaky vessels," should be easy to read as they seemingly lack the discipline men possess. Men's censure of ornamented women as lacking an authentic self denies the possibility of women exercising the same masculine control that places them on a gender parity. These men have constructed a simplistic binary to maintain their supremacy: Either women are easy to read through their bodies' external expressions of their interior passions, or they have created a public appearance devoid of an authentic self underneath. Women are either completely real or completely fake. Shamela's writings, however, undermine this simplistic gender taxonomy. She not only states her intent and ambitions clearly to the reader but also methodically demonstrates how she conducts her performance. This "behind-the-scenes" look provides insight into the real Shamela, the actress behind the role. Although, according to medical discourse, maidservants are seen as being closer in gender proximity to men, Shamela is *seen* as a woman through her gender performance of virtuous femininity. At the same time, her writing reflects an autonomous feminine identity that pushes against the gender and class ideologies of the femininity she performs.

Shamela's bodily performance demonstrates her savvy knowledge of how ideal femininity manifests on a woman's body, how a "real woman" expresses emotion through involuntary blushing. The motion of blood in a body functions as a cultural and medical signifier of femininity. As Freind writes, "How the Passion of the Mind introduces new motions into the Blood, is perhaps difficult to explain; but that they do is most certain." He explains that strong emotions trigger the "Blood to be carried on with a very rapid Motion, and that therefore it strikes against the sides of the canals with the greater impulse; which if it strike with much vehemence, the uterine vessels are easily separated."[36] When a woman suffers from suppression of the blood, the plethoric humors cause the chyle to be "more crude and viscid," resulting in a number of symptoms including pale cheeks from "the Blood being render'd thicker" and unable to "pervade the very minute Vessels in the Face."[37] This medical belief that a woman's inability to menstruate signifies bodily masculinity corresponds with the prevailing moral rhetoric of the period, which associated blushing with feminine innocence. John Donne's "Second Anniversary" praised the nonlinguistic expression of virtue of this sudden rush of blood: "her pure and eloquent blood; Spoke in her cheeks so distinctly wrought / that one might almost say, her body thought."[38] While Richard Steele in *The Spectator* (1713) commented on the ambiguity of the blush, "the livery of both guilt and innocence," both men and women celebrated the cultural ethos of the blush as a sign of attractive feminine virtue.[39] Fielding himself gives the gentle Sophia Western in *Tom Jones* this trait; she blushes when her aunt finds her reading privately and when the subject of Bliflil is brought up in conversation. But Shamela, having previously experienced carnal bliss with Parson Williams, feigns this sexual innocence on her wedding night: "In my last I left off at our sitting down to Supper on our Wedding Night, where I behaved with as much Bashfulness as the purest Virgin in the World could have done. The most difficult task for me was to blush; however, by holding my Breath, and squeezing my cheeks with my handkerchief, I did pretty well" (334). Ruth Yeazell concludes in her study of the blush in the period that "what men saw in the blushing young woman was also modesty's other face—the implicit promise of her ardent surrender."[40] When a woman blushes, her lover observes the momentary and silent yielding to her passion that would otherwise have been a secret inclination. It is unsurprising, then, that Shamela expects Booby to see her covered in anxious blushes before consummation. She recognizes the difficulty of faking a blush, but she succeeds in appearing as sexually timid as the "purest Virgin in the World." Behind the scenes, Shamela demonstrates how one can manipulate one's body to reframe existing gender and class ideologies—that a maidservant can enact virtue as well as a gentlewoman—and how much those who are participating in the discourse value bodily signifiers. In the case of the blush, it is an expression of nonlinguistic female bodily excess tinged with modest sexuality that is permissible, even encouraged.

As "leaky vessels," women's bodies involuntarily reveal their interior passions, with blushing being a prime example. It is no wonder that Richardson's use of the epistolary form best translates feminine expression, and as a consequence, he has been characterized as a "feminine" writer, with Fielding as his "masculine" contrast.[41] Fielding's use of the epistolary mode in *Shamela* plays a large role in the parody, but the use also acknowledges the epistemological value of letters in narrative truth. *Shamela* unapologetically forwards itself as a kind of exposé. Upon receiving Parson Tickletext's letter praising *Pamela*, Parson Oliver responds by sending a packet of the *true* papers of *Pamela*: "the whole Narrative is such a Misrepresentation of Facts, such a Perversion of Truth, as you will, I am perswaded, agree, as soon as you have perused the Papers I now inclose to you, that I hope you or some well-disposed Person, will communicate these Papers to the Publick, that this little Jade may not impose on the World, as she hath on her Master" (313–314). *Shamela*, then, performs the public service of correcting the "Misrepresentation of Facts" in the widely acclaimed *Pamela*, whose readership seemed to unequivocally accept her sincerity. Fielding also slightly alters the single-view narrative of *Pamela* by including corroborating evidence from other characters including her mother, Henrietta Andrews; Parson Williams; and the Lincolnshire housekeeper, Lucretia Jervis. And if the reader has somehow missed the point of Fielding's satire, Parson Oliver's final letter hammers five reasons why *Pamela* is "ridiculous" and by "no means innocent" (343). Fielding mimics Richardson's mode of storytelling but incorporates a variety of other character voices to critique the one-sided narrative as unreliable, granting the reader enough distance (rather than the harmful effects of full immersion) to discern the absurdities in Richardson's novel.

Despite *Shamela*'s multivocal approach aimed at reducing reader immersion, Shamela develops as a character beyond simple caricature as she reclaims her womanhood and selfhood through the epistolary form. Elizabeth Heckendorn Cook argues in her study of epistolary fiction that the letter represented the private, specifically "identified with the body, especially a female body, and the somatic terrain of the emotions, as well as with the thematic material of love, marriage, and the family."[42] However, epistolary fiction "exposes the private body to publication" and is both "formally and thematically concerned with competing definitions of subjectivity: it puts into play the tension between the private individual, identified with a specifically gendered, classed body that necessarily commits it to specific forms of self-interest, and the public person, divested of self-interest, discursively constituted, and functionally disembodied."[43] Shamela's status as a servant, in addition to her gender, adds further complexity to her subjectivity. If, as Robbins suggests, servant speech is audience-oriented inside interpersonal dialogue between employer and servant, and with the wider readership of the collection of letters that constitute the novella, then Shamela's "public person" has a different effect. Shamela is not divested of self-interest, as she represents underclass women and their material realities, and she is not functionally disembodied, as she actively resists individualist disembodiment from servitude.

Furthermore, Shamela's language in the epistolary mode signals the same glimpse of alternate futures, the possibility of underclass female agency that destabilizes the authority of the wealthy men who draw their power from dehumanizing women in their employ. Nicola Watson interprets the letter as a signifier of women's sexual transgression and of treason and subversion overall.[44] The content of Shamela's letters unmistakably offers evidence of her sexual transgressions. She performs "vartue" to secure financial stability with Booby while enjoying a satisfying sexual relationship with Parson Williams, going as far as making a joke at Booby's expense: "O Parson Williams, how little are all the Men in the World compared to thee" (329). But the *act* of writing such letters is also sexually transgressive. In *Pamela,* Mr. B insists that Pamela's writing is immodest, claiming that she "[gives] herself too much Licence" in his home. He worries that family secrets will be made public: "If she stays here," he warns, "she will not write the Affairs of my Family purely for an Exercise to her Pen and her Invention. . . . She is a subtle artful Gypsey."[45] Jessica L. Leiman reads Mr. B's complaint as Pamela's sexual aggression toward him: "Like the well-exercised pen that makes him so anxious, Pamela's 'licentious Tongue' seems an instrument of phallic force: both implements empower the narratives that her master suggestively calls her 'Freedoms,' 'Liberties,' 'Pertness,' and 'Boldness'—charges of class insubordination that, by design, resonate as sexual allegations as well."[46] The squire's complaint of women's writing as immodest echoes contemporary criticism against women writers such as Aphra Behn, Delarivier Manley, and Eliza Haywood.[47]

Richardson himself protests against emboldened women writers, condemning novels written by "those of the Sex" whose "loose writings . . . debauch the Mind" and who, "like the fallen Angels, having lost their own Innocence, seem, as one would think by their Writings, to make it their Study to corrupt the Minds of others, and render them as depraved, as miserable, and as lost as themselves."[48] These "loose writings" of "leaky vessels" signify unacceptable, contagious female excess from their bodies onto paper. Circulating private thoughts to a public audience, whether through personal correspondence or wider publication, is viewed as a violation of established gender boundaries, implying the masculine fear of authorial castration. Women taking narrative control enfeeble masculine voices that seek to dominate the storytelling. The self-assertion of women writers can only be read as a sexual position, as male superiority is grounded in their dominance as sexual beings. While Shamela's explicit sexuality in her letters undermines Pamela's claims to virtue, her assertion as a sexual being doubly rejects her inferior status both as a servant and as a woman. She pushes back against the virtuous, middle-class femininity embodied by Pamela, even as Shamela performs such femininity, and wrests control from the masculine vision and control of reality. And with the epistolary network of low and fellow servant women assisting Shamela in achieving her ambitions, Fielding demonstrates the extensive power of collaboration among underclass women.

### *Selfhood through Servant Community/Confederacy*

Not only does Shamela refuse disembodiment in her servitude, but she also acts as a revolutionary agent in collective effort with her mother and other servants. As leaky, underclass women, their bodily embodiment takes on a double subordination: Rebelling against the refusal of a selfhood and community solidarity, Shamela and her cohort weaponize their excess to assert autonomy and agency denied to them. As the major voice in the novella, Shamela assumes a privileged critical position alongside other laboring women. Writing to Mary Wortley Montagu, Elizabeth Carter refers to servants as "one of the most independent classes of our community," that "their covenant is founded on a reciprocation of benefit."[49] Shamela's performance of "virtue," noted by Claudio Guillén, is "the necessary dissimulation of the poor when obliged to give an account of themselves . . . to the rich and powerful."[50] Her upper-servant status as a lady's maid allows her proximity to observe and practice genteel performativity. Scarlet Bowen, in her discussion on the *Pamela* culture wars, writes that "in depicting Pamela's successful resistance to Mr. B, Richardson exploits Pamela's hybrid social identity, highlighting the strengths—artfulness, verbal assertiveness, and a practical and informed stance about sexual relations—that she derives from her position as a servant and from her connections to laboring-class femininity."[51] While anti-Pamelist texts like *Shamela* may suggest the importance of class distinctions for the maintenance of hierarchies and the justification of maidservants' exploitation, "class distinction also mattered in a somewhat progressive way in their acknowledgement of the vibrant, assertive roles of servant and laboring women."[52]

Fielding may represent Shamela's plotting as a conspiracy between underclass women, but this representation also draws attention to their spirit and boldness against a system designed to exploit them. After Shamela misreads Henrietta's warning—a caution against male perfidy, not sexual restraint—Henrietta dispenses some business advice: "When I advised you not to be guilty of Folly, I meant no more than that you should take care to be well paid before-hand, and not trust to Promises, which a Man seldom keeps, after he hath had his wicked Will" (316). In the material realities of these women's world, a man's promise is worthless. In the world of *Pamela*, the housekeepers have an ambivalent relationship with the heroine—with Mrs. Jewkes appearing as a more sinister antagonist and enabler of sexual violence—but in *Shamela*, the solidarity between servants is stronger. Shamela notes Mrs. Jervis's risky boldness toward Booby: "Mrs. Jervis made him a saucy Answer; which any Servant of Spirit, you know, would, tho' it should be one's Ruin" (319). Shamela's defense of Mrs. Jervis's impertinence as a "Servant of Spirit" is a testament to the servant woman collective that refuses to be bowed down. Mrs. Jervis reciprocates the compliment to Henrietta, writing that "Miss defended herself with great Strength and Spirit" after Booby's verbal abuse. And when Booby assumes that he has discreetly spirited Shamela away to his Lincolnshire house, his coachman Robin relays this piece of news to Mrs. Jervis, who then shares it with Henrietta. Robin was "intrusted by his Master to carry on this Affair privately," but Mrs. Jervis notes Booby's failure to realize that the household servants "hang together . . . as well as any Family of Servants in the Nation" (321). The use of the term "family" to describe the network of servants in Booby's household indicates the close bonds of social kinship between them and the collective risk they all undertake to ensure not only the safety of the vulnerable—in this case, a young maidservant—but also the stream of information necessary to execute the plan to elevate a member's social status. The servants do not view Shamela's ascent as an individual success but as a collective one. Employers like Booby, in their arrogance, underestimate servants' solidarity and overestimate servants' loyalty.

Shamela's independent spirit and generosity toward her servant brethren stand out as much more energized than Pamela's. In Richardson's rendering of the maidservant, Mr. B commands her to gift the household servants with a hundred guineas shortly after their wedding. In *Shamela*, there is no such directive from Booby, and she boldly asks for an additional hundred, which she subsequently gives away to "a Beggar," "a Man riding along the Road," and others (335). And after pressing him to give her *another* hundred, to his initial objections, she pointedly says, "[And] if you think, because I was a Servant, that I shall be contented to be governed as you please, I will shew you, you are mistaken. If you had not cared to marry me, you might have let it alone. I did not ask you, nor I did not court you" (336). While her financial security rests on her marriage to Booby, Shamela defines her selfhood independently from him. She makes it abundantly clear that he never possessed her as his servant, nor does he now as his wife. Whereas in *Pamela*, as many critics have noted, the heroine's fitness for wifehood relies on her past servitude. Terry Castle explains, "Much of the interest in [*Pamela*] . . . lies precisely in the way the heroine's private discourse—which up to a point is basically spirited and self-respecting—modulates into a fairly embarrassing political statement: a paean to womanly subjugation—marriage with the 'master.'"[53] The distinction, Nancy Armstrong writes, between "the unnatural submission of a household servant to her master in an erotic adventure" and "the natural subordination of a female to male in an ideal marriage" becomes apparent.[54] Jocelyn Harris notes that once Pamela marries, she "has little freedom "to be her own self."[55] Pamela's language after the marriage is not merely self-effacing but downright demeaning: "what is it for such a Worm as I to be exalted!" (303). And in contrast with Shamela's plans to "shew" Booby her independence in marriage, Pamela will "think [herself] more and more his servant" (257). Pamela's language almost perfectly aligns with the rhetoric in the advice book *A Present for Servants*: "that you diligently apply yourselves to know and do the Will of your Master."[56] Within the ideology of servant-employer relations, servants were considered to be the employer's property. This concept of ownership produced two conflicting traditions: the justification of an employer's right to sexually exploit maidservants and his obligations to protect them. Pamela relies on the paternalist model for her own protection and survival as a servant and continues to depend on this model to perform the duties of a submissive wife. In Armstrong's interpretation of Mr. B's sexual contract, Richardson's placement of Pamela's voice into the sphere dominated by Mr. B's contract "empowers the subject of aristocratic power with speech"; the woman is an independent party with whom the man has to negotiate, "a female self who exists outside and prior to the relationships under the male's control."[57] While Pamela resists Mr. B's sexual advances and refuses his proposal to become his mistress, she gives herself freely to him in marriage. In contrast, Shamela refuses the servant-employer ideology of servant dispossession and disembodiment. Fielding reframes her sense of feminine selfhood through her continued affiliation with other laboring women and their collective assertiveness and strength.

The confederacy of laboring women in *Shamela* has been interpreted as proof that these women are irredeemably morally inferior, corrupt, and dangerous to the social order. While *Shamela*'s central humor is at Booby's expense, the alternate world in which laboring women hold power serves as an expression of the real fear of social upheaval. Fielding's conservative agenda in favor of a strict social hierarchy is clear, and the burlesque's ending contains any sustained momentum for change. In Parson Tickletext's final postscript, Shamela and Parson Williams receive their comeuppance: "Mr. Booby hath caught his Wife in bed with Williams; hath turned her off, and is prosecuting him in the spiritual Court" (344). Ultimately, Fielding reprimands these expressions of laboring women's sexual and self-assertiveness. *Shamela*'s humor gives its audience the feminist fantasy of revolutionary possibility, whether that fantasy provokes anxiety or hope, only to ultimately reinforce the conservative power structures that were momentarily subverted.

## *HUMPHRY CLINKER*

While Shamela embodies underclass empowerment through bodily performance, Winifred Jenkins in *Humphry Clinker* asserts a similar subversive power through her writing. Her malapropisms, Smollett's literary burlesque of underclass literacy, represent the leaky female body and reposition this body in a celebratory light, offering a counterdiscourse to conservative attitudes about servant literacy. This representation of the Welsh maid's authentic speech patterns of her class allows her to reclaim ownership of her language; she assumes power through the narrative and gains autonomy over the text's meaning through the rhythms of her community's speech patterns. Win's language recasts the negative portrayal of underclass women as sexually and linguistically intemperate. Rather, her linguistic intemperance focuses the positive materiality of her speech through her underclass female body, becoming an expression of fertility, bounty, and potentiality outside her employer's dominance.

In *Humphry Clinker*, regarded as Smollett's finest novel, Win's writing has been typically viewed as one long joke on underclass illiteracy. Robert D. Spector notes that Win serves as the "object of humor in Smollett's class-conscious audience."[58] The novel is composed of a series of letters written by members of the Bramble family that document their experiences and reflections on their tour through England and Scotland. Prone to folk expressions and mangling words that result in puns and double entendre, Win's entries have long been considered as the major source of comic energy in the novel.[59] Esther K. Sheldon praises Smollett's crafting of Win's language, describing it as a "pleasant source of humor throughout the book," and she says that, though it is a bit on the scatological side, it is "a bright thread throughout the story."[60] Austin Dobson, a nineteenth-century literary critic, places Win among the most memorable comic characters of the preceding century: "Not even the Malapropism of Sheridan or Dickens is quite as riotously diverting, as rich in its unexpected turns, as that of Tabitha Bramble and Winifred Jenkins, especially Winifred, who remains delightful even when deduction is made of the poor and very mechanical fun extracted from the parody of her pietistic phraseology."[61] Through Win's language, Smollett has crafted comic carnivalesque speech to perfection. Despite the humor's crudeness, which frequently returns to bodily functions improper for polite discourse, readers find Win to be charming, likeable, and frankly, more memorable than the other female characters in the novel. Furthermore, her writing and speech provide an alternate discourse within the novel's heteroglot landscape that gives legitimacy to the lived experiences of the underclass.

Smollett's artistic sensibilities and convictions as a failed physician often converged in his representation of the human body.[62] Before writing novels, Smollett's first break into the literary world was in the theater, an art form reliant on both physical and auditory expression. Like his predecessor Fielding, Smollett's interest in the theater greatly influenced his prose. Reminiscent of Hogarth's caricatures, the episodic orientation of his novels arrests characters and space in striking illustration. Critics have recognized this rich texture of Smollett's intensely physical portraits. Besides George S. Rousseau's exploration on the novel's medical background, David Weed's reading finds a resisting masculinity in an infectious and feminine commercialism through Matt Bramble's journey to health.[63] Aileen Douglas's work focuses on Smollett's interest with the human body and its cultural significance.[64] John McAllister's work on symptomatology and the representation of character elucidates Smollett's reliance on contemporary medical assumptions about the physical manifestations of human emotion.[65] I expand on these investigations of the novel's medical themes in the context of Win's carnivalesque language and its relationship to medical representations of menstruation and female excess.

### *Humor and the Humors*

Excess in Win's speech patterns, embodied most clearly in her embarrassing outbursts and exclamations, frequently parodies other medical phenomena. Clinker, a servant whom Matthew Bramble picked up en route and who becomes Win's love interest, has been falsely accused of robbery. In Win's letter to her fellow maidservant Mary Jones, she declares, "the whole family has been in such a constipation!"[66] Win's confusing "consternation" with "constipation" produces a joke at the maidservant's expense, but this humorous substitution carries greater significance than mere wordplay. Both words share meaning within the context of eighteenth-century medical thought, which was still rooted in the humoral framework that had dominated early modern medical scholarship.[67] According to this model, the black bile, one of the four humors, becomes aggravated through prolonged stress. This inflammation would lead to an accumulation of excess bile, or plethora, in the bowels and lower digestive tract, resulting in constipation. The eminent Dutch physician Herman Boerhaave recognized this psychosomatic event in his *Aphorisms* (1728), a textbook compendium of disease and treatment. Melancholy, for example, "begin[s] in what is called the Mind" and "doth render the Choler black in the Body very soon."[68] The thickening of blood, also called "melancholy juice," results in symptoms of "constant Weight, Anguish, Fullness" that include "Belches, Winds, Cramps, Costiveness and very hard Stools."[69] Séverine Pilloud and Micheline Louis-Courvoisier note that author-physicians "in studying the influence of the passions on human organization have observed that . . . the sad passions, like grief, boredom and fear, almost always appear in the abdominal organs."[70] The family's anxiety during Clinker's trial, as Win mentions, may have caused someone to experience melancholic excess from pathologized black bile. The family head, Matt Bramble, who suffered from chronic gastrointestinal discomfort, confesses as much to his doctor: "The imprisonment of Clinker brought on those symptoms which I mentioned in my last [letter], and now they are vanished at his discharge" (146). The reader would not have missed the comic wordplay of "discharge" for Clinker's release and Matthew's digestive relief. This example demonstrates the inextricable relationship between humor and the body in *Humphry Clinker*'s sustained scatological elements.

Smollett's crafting of Win's writing style exemplifies both bodily and linguistic excess and loss of restraint in distinctly female terms. In a letter dated June 3, she recounts her dizzying first experience with London:

> O Molly! What shall I say of London! All the towns that ever I beheld in my born-days, are no more than Welsh barrows and crumlecks to this wonderful sitty! Even Bath itself is but a fillitch, in the naam of God—one would think there's no end of the streets, but the land's end. Then there's such a power of people, going hurry skurry! Such a racket of coxes! Such a noise and haliballoo! So many strange sites to be seen! O gracious! My poor Welsh brain has been spinning like a top ever since I came hither! And I have seen the Park, and the paleass of Saint Gimses, and the king's and the queen's magisterial pursing, and the sweet young princes, and the hilly-fents, and pye-bald ass, and all the rest of the royal family. (101–102)

Win's series of amazed exclamations pour out of her, with her "poor Welsh brain" unable to absorb the exhilarating sights of London with restraint. The stream of conjunctions in the last sentence listing the sights at St. James's Palace replicates the sensory overload experienced by a tourist navigating the bustling chaos of London. While cultural and scientific discourse marks the female body as a leaky vessel incapable of self-government, placing the male above in the hierarchy of bodily self-rule, the unbridled expressiveness in Win's writing repudiates the negative inscriptions associated with womanhood. The servant's language articulates the tensions between the intellectual elite and the disenfranchised by parodying the woman's hemorrhaging body represented as weaker and inferior in medical texts such as Freind's. Here, literary burlesque configured in the porous and fluid Bakhtinian body empowers Win's agency, both as an underclass writer and as a woman. Menstrual cycles cannot be controlled, yet they serve as a measure of women's health and fertility, an advantage for the humoral diagnosis and treatment of women. Win's prose reveals a bodily life that is fertile and abundant, exemplary of the Bakhtinian grotesque. Bakhtin explains, "the very material bodily lower stratum of the grotesque image (food, wine, the genital force, the organs of the body) bears a deeply positive character" in reflecting the universal, the people, materializing the abstract and the ideal into flesh.[71] Win's free and frank expressions resonate with the Bakhtinian marketplace, where all talk surpasses verbal limitations and conventions. Read this way, the narrative's dialogic force renders these verbal limitations absolutely relative and crystallizes Win's writing as a concrete heteroglot expression of the people's world, offered through images of the leaky feminine body.

## *Compulsory Fluency and the Grotesque*

Smollett stylizes Win's language for readers to inhabit her own realities as an underclass woman, and the crucial features of this stylization are the phonetic, grammatical, and syntactical divergences. Her writing deviates from standard grammatical and orthographic norms, creating a grotesque image of language. For example, writing from Bath, she reports to Molly receiving her mistress's "yallow trollopea" and how much the color flatters her complexion: "You knows as how, yallow fitts my fizzogmony" (40). Yellow, a color that signals a choleric temperament resulting from an excess of yellow bile, corresponds with Win's immoderation in both personality and irregular writing style. Many of Smollett's predecessors commented on the regularity of English spelling. Critics like Joseph Addison and Richard Steele frequently turned to the subject in satirical pieces in *The Spectator* and *The Tatler*; Daniel Defoe discusses the problem at length in *The Compleat English Gentleman* (1728); and Jonathan Swift wrote most notably on the issue in his *Proposal for Correcting, Improving and Ascertaining the English Tongue* (1712).[72] And Thomas Sheridan, in his influential *Dissertation on the Causes of the Difficulties, Which Occur, in Learning of the English Tongue* (1762), placed a nationalist imperative on standardizing speech and writing rules to create a homogenized, unified Britain loyal to its imperial ambitions: The "attainment of the English tongue in its purity, both in print of phraseology and pronunciation, might be rendered easy to all inhabitants of his Majesty's dominions, whether of South or North Brittain; of Ireland or the Colonies."[73] Jared S. Richman remarks that Sheridan's attention to the "purity" of "the English tongue" "should not only give us pause for the way in which it privileges an ideal (in this case, normative) manner of speaking, but also for codifying a category of deviant speech into which all other phraseologies and pronunciations must necessarily fall. The demand for vocal purity casts a stigma of immorality upon those unwilling or, more troublingly, unable to conform linguistically."[74] Richman calls this mandate "compulsory fluency" in theorizing how disabled elocution operated as a governing trope in Georgian Britain: "Compulsory fluency becomes a powerful mechanism for a British nationalism that is predicated on a model of disability casting individual non-normative speakers as morally suspect, socially deviant, and politically irrelevant."[75] Although (as far as we know) Winifred is not disabled, Richman's framing of compulsory fluency is useful in explaining how gender and class can also violate emerging linguistic social norms, especially within the context of the medical model that determined women as unable to self-regulate. The materiality of speech is inextricable from embodiment and could stand for nonnormative bodies.

Linguistic difference, therefore, materializes on the page and draws attention to the ways in which the intersections of gender and class are marked on underclass women's bodies as aberrant. The rising cultural imperative for compulsory fluency would then require distinctions of otherness to uphold the hierarchy of normalization. Win's otherness, especially among the other letter writers who conform more closely to grammatical and orthographic norms, becomes more pronounced. And in the context of the eighteenth century, as Lennard Davis has noted, the construction of "normalcy" is the "political-juridical-institutional state that relies on the control and normalization of bodies."[76] Any deviation from normalcy, Essaka Joshua explains, could be construed as deformity, signifying a visual, observable atypicality in a person's corporeal constitution, without necessarily indicating a physical impairment.[77] And considering how women are conceptualized under the category of deformity, Helen Deutsch and Felicity Nussbaum argue that women's bodily difference is analogous to deformity or monstrosity; women are essentially defective.[78] Introducing the intersectional category of class, servant women like Win, whose abnormally menstruating bodies are medically conceptualized to be distinctly more masculine or genderfluid compared to their genteel employers, are doubly further removed from the norm. This double deformity is made manifest in Win's writing style.

Of all the senses affected by the grotesque, sight is the one most severely offended. Lennard Davis writes, "Rather than disability, what is called to readers' attention before the eighteenth century is deformity, . . . a disruption in the sensory field of the observer."[79] Subject to laughter, the deformed body's visibly exaggerated character degrades the ideal. This degradation is comically illustrated with Win praying often for "God's grease" (204). The misspelling of "grace," the favor of God as manifested in the salvation of sinners and the bestowal of blessings, undercuts the divine association by the corporeal association of "grease," or rendered animal fat. The spiritual is transformed into the material entity of writing. In other words, Smollett's burlesque of the servant's language reifies what Bakhtin calls "grotesque realism," transforming deformity from a punch line to an open challenge against the legitimacy of existing structural power relations. Win's difference, materialized in her writing style, embodies the spirit of humor and chaos that subverts and questions the normative assumptions of dominant culture.

Despite the devaluation of "grace," the grotesque in the comic, written here as "grease," gestures to the body's positive force. Bakhtin finds the "deeply positive" aspect of the grotesque body in its degradation—defined in its needs for eating, drinking, having sex, defecating—by linking it to birth and renewal.[80] Medical discourse, however, inscribed women's bodies in a constant state of unhealthiness, a biological burden they must accept and carry. In the case of menstruation, physicians such as Freind viewed this bodily function as evidence of the woman's lifelong vulnerability to illness and suffering. Paradoxically, in relation to men's health, the assessment of women's physical well-being depends on the degree of how unhealthy she is not. Since women's bodies leaked, they were inscribed with weakness and loss of control, in contrast to the robust masculine body that exercised bourgeois principles of self-possession:

> Wretched surely and unequal seems the condition of the Female Sex, that they who are by Nature destined to be the Preservers of the Human Race, should at the same time be made liable to so many Diseases. For whatever Course of Life they pursue, few there are, who enjoy an Health untainted and exempt from Pain: for if they enter into a wedded State, even from that source of Pleasures something bitter arises, and Pregnancy brings with it at least a length of loathing, if nothing more calamitous; if they make a Vow of Celibacy, wite all their precaution they will hardly be able to avoid labouring under some Distemper, even upon that very account, because they are strangers to a Mother's Pangs. For that supply of Blood which Women ought to collect for the use and aliment of their Offspring, if it either inwardly increase, or flow something immoderately, excites a thousand Disorders in their tender Frame.[81]

Women, whose bodies evacuate excess of fluid, are doomed to be "wretched" since they are housed in a "tender frame."

Although menstruation signified negative perceptions of womanhood, marking bodies according to class or gender, Win's free and sincere expressions negate this negative femininity and social caste. The grotesque realism of Win's servant writing rejuvenates the linguistic system in the novel and allows for progress in the novel's democratic approach to underclass literacy. I find that the novel's comic mode exhibits the grotesque body of writing in celebrating an alternative literacy instead of merely satirizing the rudimentary efforts of underclass people to read and write. Information on early literacy continues to be far from definitive, but important work by J. Paul Hunter and Jan Fergus suggests that servants read or were exposed to reading material by their literate employers and peers.[82] Conduct manuals, sermons, and pamphlets codified appropriate reading behavior for servants, indicating a cultural anxiety surrounding servant literacy.[83] Writers worried that reading could mislead people in the lower orders in their expectations about life, corrupt their reasoning in valuing sentiment over rationality, and overheat the passions in inflaming their imaginations. Judith Frank observes, "along with women and apprentices, servants stood at the boundary of the literacy/nonliteracy divide, and as such were a particular source of anxiety to the eighteenth-century ruling class, which was acutely aware of the ideology-forming powers of the printed word."[84] As the number of literate domestic servants grew, writers became increasingly conscious of how the text could impact moral character. Despite this cultural uneasiness of underclass literacy, the comic novel's inclusion of the grotesque, with its emphasis on the body, presents a counterdiscourse to conservative attitudes.

In the substitution of "grace" with "grease," which recalls Shamela's "vartue," the grotesque image materializes the ideal into the flesh through writing, linking composition with human anatomy. This body-centric writing articulates the social history of physiology and comic language. The Third Earl of Shaftesbury viewed the deformed body as a form of moral transgression: "Natural health is the just proportion, truth, and regular course of things in a constitution. It is the inward beauty of the body. And when the harmony and just measures of the rising pulses, the circulating humours, and the moving airs or spirits, are disturbed or lost, deformity enters, and with it, calamity and ruin."[85] The deformed body not only raised suspicion of moral character but also became the subject of ridicule. In addition to these suspicions, critics of eighteenth-century humor note that the English had a long-standing tradition of laughing at deformity and handicap.[86] In Simon Dickie's study of mid-eighteenth-century jestbooks that targeted dwarfs, cripples, and hunchbacks, he interprets these texts as suggesting "an almost unquestioned pleasure at the sight of deformity or misery. . . . Any deformity or incapacity was infallibly, almost instinctively, amusing."[87] From these two perspectives, the body was thought to be the material expression of moral character or virtue. Its disfigurement, or the grotesque figure of the body, often invoked laughter. The analogy between the deformed or grotesque body and burlesqued writing lies in their material and concrete manifestations. Both images, one of a person and another of a language, represent the irregular, the imperfect, the distorted. Both images are available visually to the viewer. Both images also elicit the same somatic response: laughter. In this way, burlesqued writing is intimately linked with the body.

The carnivalesque materializes in Win's writing when she describes her bath in Loch Lomond during the family's stay in "Haddingborrough," following the advice of the local witch to cure her of her "fits" (242). Win ingenuously believes the myth that a "musician" created the reputedly bottomless lake, as she sees no other explanation for the "waves without wind, fish without fins, and [the] floating hyland" (241). While bathing with a fellow maid in this legendary body of water, Sir George Colquhoun, Matt's guide in the Scottish Highlands, spies the two women in their "birthday-soot" (242). For Win and her fellow maidservant, the term's distortion from nudity to "soot," a substance that coats maidservants during their duties in tending fireplaces, invokes not only the body but also their social status. This demarcation of gender is also present in Smollett's earlier novel *The Adventures of Ferdinand Count Fathom* (1753), in which there is a stark contrast in bodily constitutions between women and men. When the major receives the hero at the door "in cuerpo," "he made an apology for receiving the Count in his birthday suit, to which he said he was reduced by the heat of his constitution."[88] Corresponding with humoral belief, this "Herculean" soldier's extreme warmth, matching his warlike passion evidenced by his proud display of battle scars to Fathom, characterizes his body as robustly masculine. While the major's nude body celebrates the masculine, the maidservants' nudity suggests both the feminine and the underclass in the malaprose. To a larger extent, soot signifies the wretched conditions of the laboring class; many chimney sweepers and their young apprentices suffered debilitating long-term effects to their health from inhaling the toxic material.[89] Win's literacy fuses gender and status, disrupting the novel's conventional narrative style and the reader's imagination. Considering the liberating and disruptive qualities of low humor, Smollett's configuration of servant writing in burlesque animates the novel's linguistic landscape with carnivalesque energy.

It is significant, then, that Win's writing introduces chaos into the structured realm of "correct language." Smollett stylizes her language with puns, playing with sounds that create meanings only available in the servant's burlesqued writing. These puns, in turn, cause confusion and impede understanding, acting as an anarchic force in the system of linguistic order. Correct language, or what Bakhtin terms "common unitary language," is a system of linguistic standards, including grammatical and spelling conventions, and universal syntactical principles that writers like Swift and Defoe campaigned for in their writings. Bakhtin does not view correct language as inexorably authoritative; rather, these norms create generative energy that engages with the other voices in heteroglossia, seeking either to "centralize" one official language or to defend such language from a continually expanding heteroglossia.[90] Low language, exemplified in the servant's writing, critiques the notion of any centralized linguistic system. The artistic rendering of servant literacy in the grotesque exposes the myths in medical discourse. This suggests that comic language, metaphorically imagined here as representing the leaky female body in grotesque writing, affirms the political legitimacy of low and gendered language in the novel's linguistic tapestry.

In a brilliant moment of self-reflexive humor, Win promotes servant literacy in a letter dated June 3. As an example of "low genre," Win's writing sharply parodies literary language: "And I pray of all love, you will mind your vriting and your spilling; for, craving your pardon, Molly, it made me suet to disseyfer your last scrabble, which was delivered by the hind at Bath—O, voman! Voman! If thou had'st but the least consumption of what pleasure we scullers have, when we can cunster the crabbidst buck off hand, and spell ethnitch vords without lucking at the primmer" (103). Win calling herself a "sculler" instead of a "scholar" opens a multiplicity of meanings. This deliberate emphasis on physical rather than intellectual labor classifies Win's language and character as distinctly underclass. Though Smollett's own *Critical Review* regarded the uncontrolled spread of reading as a social menace, the configuration of servant literacy, reified in grotesque materialism, mocks conventional language and mirrors the chaotic linguistic panorama of the novel.[91] Win closes the letter with "yours with true infection," suggesting the communicable nature of servant literacy through correspondence and social support.

And truly, the strength of the servant community's bonds enabled access to literacy. Though a small minority of servants were formally educated, all servants were exposed to a considerable amount of literature, namely, through the male head of the household or sometimes the mistress, reading aloud sermons or other bits of morally edifying literature, especially the Bible.[92] Servants also had access to their employer's library and could purchase cheaper pirated copies or chapbooks of popular works.[93] Jan Fergus suggests that servants were a fair proportion of literate individuals by the middle of the century, and they preferred a range of fiction, especially drama, in their literary choices.[94] In light of the growth of print culture in the eighteenth century, John Brewer notes, "Books, print and readers were everywhere. Not everyone was a reader, but even those who could not read lived to an unprecedented degree in a culture of print, for the impact of the publishing revolution extended beyond the literate."[95] Adam Fox investigates the interplay of orality and literacy in England and argues that written texts, in the form of scandalous ballads and humorous verses familiarized by the people, were sustained and transformed by their connection with other activities like singing, narrating, and listening.[96] Communal activities engaged the illiterate with literacy, and the term "reading community" resounds very strongly for servants, as their experience in literacy relied on the collective act of reading, listening, and recitation.[97] Even if individuals in the lower ranks of society were not given formal scribal training, as their more genteel counterparts received private tutoring as children, elements of print culture were available to them as a group. For eighteenth-century servants, literacy encompassed a broader spectrum than modern audiences might understand. To this end, Smollett's "double-voicing" of the maidservant character in linguistic excess and physical obscenity exerts a revolutionizing influence on any kind of normative linguistics of the novel.

For Bakhtin, "the symbols of the carnival idiom are filled with [the] pathos of change and renewal, with the sense of the gay relativity of prevailing truths and authorities."[98] To simply regard Win's writing as the scribblings of an illiterate servant whose misspellings and malapropisms exist solely for comic effect would diminish Smollett's greatest, most richly rendered novel. The plenitude of meanings opened from these orthographic errors attests to the fullness of linguistic grotesque realism that collapses the body and writing. Win's servant literacy, stylized in low humor, asserts the politically subversive quality of language in the comic novel, unsettling broader gender, status, and medical hierarchies. The novel's last entry, authored by Win, serves as Smollett's fullest and deepest expression of the ultimately protean nature of language: "Providinch hath bin pleased to make great halteration in the pasture of our affairs" (322).

## CONCLUSION

The comic representations of female underclass excess in *Shamela* and *Humphry Clinker* drew inspiration from existing medical theories about menstruation. The intersection of class and gender in Shamela's and Win's subjectivity creates a complex and sometimes contradictory convergence of oppression. As women capable of menstruation, their uncontrollable leakiness indicated their inability to govern their bodies and, by extension, themselves, requiring patriarchal regulation to protect both themselves and the social order. And yet, as servants, these women are drawn as more masculine or genderfluid, introducing a discomfiting anxiety safely contained within the comic mode. This intersectionality manifests in the double deformity in their style of writing, a kind of grotesque realism, their literacy expressing their sexual and emotional leakiness with physical obscenity that draws attention to their corporeality. The conflicting presence of the grotesque and the deformed in the comic create tension in which the grotesque pushes back against systems of domination through humor and ridicule, while the casting of deformity attempts to reinforce the normative mechanisms of those systems. Through the epistolary form, print rendered their bodies more visible and more vulnerable to critique and satire. But in the comic mode, the language of the maidservant decentralizes the male-controlled narratives that negatively show her as intemperate. Like menstruation, the servant maid's linguistic intemperance conveys abundance and possibility, asserting an independent selfhood and underclass community solidarity from their employers, who seek to empty and separate her from both.

In contrast to Richardson's Pamela, Shamela's skill in performing the virtuous bourgeois female body for her own designs (to gain access to wealth through marriage while still maintaining her sexual relationship with Parson Williams) challenges the very performativity of such underclass virtue that eventually rewards Pamela with a husband. Feigning a fainting fit and blushes to signal leisure-class delicacy and Christian chastity, reinforced by medical theories of how women's blood flowed, Shamela performs an ideal femininity that dupes her employer into an offer of marriage. And through this performance, which she makes clear in her writing, Shamela undermines both taxonomies of class and gender, ridiculing the flimsiness of both constructs on which the social order rests. What is more, Shamela's refusal of disembodiment also manifests in her agency in her marriage, as a member of the community of servants collaborating for their material success. Servant women's bodily embodiment acquires a double subordination in weaponizing excess to assert class and gender agency within systems of domination.

Similarly, Winifred's comical malapropisms, Smollett's burlesque of underclass literacy, reposition the servant maid body as imbued with a life of her own.

Her particular speech patterns, replicated in her writing's orthography, offer a counterdiscourse against the normative speech embodied by her employers in the novel that legitimizes the lived experience of the underclass. Her outbursts and exclamations convey linguistic excess and loss of restraint. This literary burlesque configured in the porous and leaky body empowers Win's agency and independence. While menstrual cycles cannot be controlled, they serve as a measure of health and fertility. It is in this excess and uncontrol that a fertile and abundant bodily life is revealed, exemplary of the Bakhtinian grotesque. Win's writing deviates from emerging grammatical and orthographic standards, creating a grotesque image of language through the framing of compulsory fluency. Win's defiance of these linguistic norms stands for her nonnormative body, illustrating how the materiality of speech is indivisible from embodiment. Her difference, as a woman and as a servant, becomes more pronounced, and this double deformity manifests in her writing style. Smollett's burlesque of servant language makes concrete what Bakhtin identifies as grotesque realism, transforming deformity from a joke into a critique of structural power relations that rely on class and gender to reinforce hierarchy. In this way, difference is expressed through this spirit of humor and upheaval.

Both maidservants, through their linguistic intemperance, assert relative agency that begins to imagine a future liberated from oppressive systems. Each, however, meets a different end: Shamela's schemes and sexual indiscretions are discovered, leading to her downfall from the position of power she had achieved through exogamous marriage, while Win is rewarded with a marriage to Humphry Clinker, a fellow servant. Both conclusions align with the comic tradition in distinct ways. While female excess is represented for comic effect through wordplay, burlesque, or raillery, it can also function as the subject of comic irony. Shamela, who is such a target due to her aspirations for social mobility through deception, needs to be knocked down to secure the happiness of more deserving characters. Who this deserving character might be in *Shamela* is unclear, but the maidservant aping her betters to climb the social ladder is cast as the wicked figure who faces punishment in the end. Fielding plays with the confusion and transgression engendered by the maidservant's leakiness, yet he returns to the conservative ending that restores domestic harmony by removing the threat to social order. Shamela's affectation embodies a femininity that is dangerous to class hierarchy and threatens contamination of the family lineage with the blood of the lowborn. Win's affectation, on the other hand, is perceived as charming in its innocuousness to the family pedigree. The world of the comic may be briefly disrupted, but the ending ultimately reaffirms the order of things. While low and gendered language within the panorama of the comic novel is acknowledged and legitimized, that is as progressive as the comic will go. Identity affirmation is allowed, but access to material wealth, reserved only for the women's employers, remains too radical for Fielding and Smollett.

In chapter 2, I continue my focus on female expression and embodiment within the context of the discourse of hysteria in Fielding's other comic novels *Tom Jones* and *Joseph Andrews*. The comic representations of the desiring female libertines Ladies Booby and Bellaston raise the same questions regarding the cultural and medical construction of gender and interrogate the promise of domestic happiness associated with living a sexually virtuous life.

2

# HYSTERICAL LANGUAGE AND DESIRING WOMEN IN HENRY FIELDING'S *JOSEPH ANDREWS* (1742) AND *TOM JONES* (1749)

THE WANTON WOMAN APPEARS AS a familiar archetype in the broad landscape of Henry Fielding's novels. These representations of female carnal excess, realized in the characters of Mrs. Slipslop in *Joseph Andrews* (1742), Jenny Jones in *Tom Jones* (1749), and Miss Matthews in *Amelia* (1751), serve as foils to the bourgeois feminine ideal that the heroines embodied. Nina Prytula categorizes these women as "Amazons . . . who attempt to subjugate the men around them by means of sheer physical (and often sexual) domination."[1] Mary Hamilton's queerness in *The Female Husband* (1746) is the extreme instance of a woman usurping masculine power.[2] However, Fielding's satire alongside coexisting medical discourse both supports and contradicts his moralist critique of female licentiousness. These women, and Fielding himself, participate in and call into question the social and medical debate of frustrated female sexual desire. In particular, the problem of women's sexual excitability and excesses pervaded discourses on hysteria. As I explained in chapter 1, women's leaky, fragile bodies signified their inability to regulate themselves. This idea extended to their emotional embodiment, suggesting that any attempt to control desire was futile since their body's vascular and reproductive mechanics left them unequipped to do so. Physicians believed that hysterical symptoms could be prevented if women accepted their place as wives and mothers; therefore, consistent sex with their husbands and ensuing pregnancies were prescribed as cures. Women's rejection of such treatments, an act of sexual self-determination, was regarded as pathological rebellion that only exacerbated their symptoms. Desiring or having sex outside of marriage was described as a manifestation of hysteric tendencies. The ways in which women's bodies were conceived as naturally incapable of physical (and, by extension, emotional and rational) self-governance make visible the gendered limitations of the Enlightenment ethos of an autonomous self. And yet, to some degree, Fielding expressed ambivalence about the healthiness (or even possibility) of absolute, unrestrained passion. Fielding underscores this problem in *Tom Jones* with passion personified as an irrepressible female intruder: "if we shut Nature out at the Door, she will come in at the Window."[3]

Fielding's gendering of nature as "she" reveals parallels in the power dynamics between male scientists and nature in similar terms between men and women: Carolyn Merchant's *Death of Nature* demonstrates that nature's scientific study has been long imagined as female, and Evelyn Fox Keller identifies science's gender as masculine in the female/nature and male/science binaries that structures the discipline's central metaphor.[4] This metaphor registers, in a great degree, the ideological underpinnings of the patriarchal institutions, including medicine, that determine and enforce normative codes of female conduct: to know and master nature and women for their potential erotic wildness as feminine sites for masculine conquest. Tita Chico reexamines gender's place in scientific subjectivity, particularly in regard to women: "By observing gender while simultaneously observing matters of literary knowledge and science, we can glimpse the wider social, ideological, and imaginative structures taking shape and coming to determine what experience, evidence, and authority could be in the British Enlightenment—including for and by whom."[5] The comic novel's interest in scientific subjectivity is made clear in the cultural anxieties toward female bodies, bodies their sexual capacity defined. Masculine conquest of these bodies takes the form of pathologizing female desire, with the cultural and medical mandate of heterosexual marriage and monogamous sex as cure.

This chapter examines the early eighteenth-century discourse on hysteria, a medical language fraught with anxieties over female sexuality and agency, and its parodic representations in *Joseph Andrews* and *Tom Jones*. I read the emotional expressions of two libertine women, Lady Booby and Lady Bellaston, who embody aristocratic license and licentiousness as sites of negotiations between medical knowledge, literature, and sexual politics in eighteenth-century culture. I refer to these expressions as "hysterical," as they resemble the features of hysteria that eighteenth-century male physicians described; uttered in the throes of unfulfilled desire, these expressions of female sexual excitability follow the epistemologies of Enlightenment medicine to passion that underscores female frailty. In chapter 1, I argued that Fielding's and Smollett's comic representations of female underclass excess drew from eighteenth-century medical theories about menstruation, producing contradictions, confusion, and anxieties regarding linguistic and sexual intemperance. In this chapter, I continue to explain how class status can determine women's embodiment in medical discourse as I shift my focus to women higher in the social hierarchy. Yet again, as it was with Shamela and Win, women's excess is perceived as a cultural problem worked through the woman's bodily operations. And again, the cure for the problems caused by this excess, seen as harmful to the woman herself, is to submit to her subordinate place.

Like Shamela's comic yet threatening pretensions for social ascent, Lady Booby's and Lady Bellaston's masculine assertions of sexual agency outside of marriage are represented as comically incongruent with social expectations. And like Shamela, their excesses serve as subjects of comic irony requiring correction through humiliation. Ladies Booby and Bellaston, driven by sexual excess, also operate as the agents impeding the happiness of more deserving characters, including the sexually demure women who are rewarded with marriage. While Lady Booby and Lady Bellaston are drawn as villains in varying degrees, I argue that the hysteric expressions of unfulfilled desire by these libertine women reveal the authentic suffering experienced by women commanded to abide by the oppressive standards of feminine virtue. Although Fielding condemns this kind of female licentiousness as detrimental to social order, he also acknowledges the emotional wretchedness that their status imposes on them.

Recent work in the humanities on "the affective turn" reconceptualizes old binary models of the opposition of reason/science and emotion/art as converging to give shape to the eighteenth-century experience.[6] Thomas Dixon argues, "The debate about the proper relationship of reason with the passions, sentiments and affections was one of the characteristic concerns of eighteenth-century thought."[7] Philosophers such as Francis Hutcheson, David Hume, Adam Smith, and John Locke conceived of the passions as more public than private, a social experience that shared principles of virtue secured; these figures tried to understand how the passions shaped public structures and how controlling those passions would direct an ordered society. The novel offered an alternative discourse of the passions in its philosophical analysis of feeling.[8] In looking at female characters' emotional lives, we see how cultural expectations of rigid virtue and the greater medical discourse that repeatedly determines the essential frailty of women's bodies to practice this virtue result in emotional, bodily, and existential distress. Women's emotional expressions of unfulfilled desire are ultimately entangled with the discourse of hysteria, for both are rooted in the mechanics of the passions and the body's inability in managing emotions. And as amatory fiction, especially Eliza Haywood's work, engages in feeling and the body, it is an especially fertile space to examine how authentic emotional representations are shaped by the discourse of hysteria in the female characters' failure to meet the standards of self-possession. Fielding harnesses amatory fiction's language both to deploy humor and to authentically represent his female characters' emotional lives.

Hysteria functioned as a cultural metaphor that articulated and confirmed women's inherent pathology; frailty, volatility, and inferior intelligence were commonly linked to women's rebellion against domesticity.[9] Sabine Arnaud claims in her study of hysteria as a medical category that writings on sexual desire as a source of hysteria marked a new significance in the 1730s.[10] Examining the discourse of hysteria, then, is uniquely relevant to reading desiring women in Fielding's novels. Through these two libertine women, the novels suggest an alternate reaction to androcentric codes of feminine modesty, one in which a natural but prohibited desire "naturally [seeks] vent" without resorting to marriage as a remedy for women in the eighteenth century. Theorists of hysteria in the period often considered the institution of marriage in their detailing of the disease since semen had a palliative effect on the turbulent womb; practitioners viewed widows, virgins, and nuns as most vulnerable to hysteria, women without access to the conjugal, and ostensibly health, benefits of a husband's semen. So strong was this belief that the most popular prescription for hysteria was marriage. Practitioners viewed women's rebellion against prescriptive domesticity as "symptoms" of self-inflicted hysteria; Guenter Risse notes that for eighteenth-century practitioners, hysterical symptoms were a "just punishment for non-conforming females who dared weaken their already fragile nerves or flaunted their sexuality."[11] Glen Colburn notes that the discourse of hysteria is rife with self-contradictions that come from writers' efforts to blend moral and physiological fact: "Because hysteria was conceived of as a psychosomatic disorder, it involved physicians in speculations about the mental, emotional, and moral as well as physical states of their patients. In other words, treatises about hysteria tend to blur the distinction between medical and moral inquiries."[12] Practitioners framed hysteria, then, as a disorder that can be prevented if women submit to the conventional gender hierarchy. If they do suffer from hysteria, symptoms will disappear once they accept their place. Both Lady Booby and Lady Bellaston, widow and single woman, respectively, recognize the oppressiveness of marriage. Subjected to both their undisciplined physiology and patriarchal institutions, their yearning for extramarital love and desire is articulated through their hysterical speech and writing.

## THE PROGRESS OF VIOLENCE IN WOMEN'S PASSIONS

Critics regard *Joseph Andrews*' Lady Booby as a negative representation of the feminine.[13] But the novel's engagement with the direct changes in social reality—cultural transformations that ushered in the modern era defined by sentimental heterosexual ethics, as described by Paul Kelleher—invites a deeper sensitivity to and reflection of linguistic flexibility.[14] Fielding's casting of female actors in male libertine roles appears to disrupt the order of power that sex categories defined, but the comic mode and the prevailing medical discourse design a world in which these women pose no real threat. In invoking the discourse of the nerve as a touchstone in his time and parodying the language of the amatory novel that Haywood popularized, writing he later deemed "foolish" and "monstrous" in the opening chapter of book 9 in *Tom Jones* (422), Fielding stages the limitations of this disruption in the essentialized representations of women as embodied beings.

Lady Booby's unhappiness exemplifies the failure of the sexual promises of matrimony. Once widowed, she makes her desires plain in the unwanted sexual advances on her attractive, young footman, Joseph. After publishing *Shamela*, Fielding continues his critique of *Pamela* with *Joseph Andrews* in wider panorama. Fielding substitutes *Pamela*'s reformed rake Mr. B with his sister, Lady Booby, and the virtuous servant maid Pamela with her brother, Joseph. This reversal seems to continue Mr. Booby's caricature in *Shamela* as a dupe of aristocratic privilege and libidinousness. However, Lady Booby's state as a rich widow with a public, independent place in patriarchal society significantly reframes the power dynamics of gender beyond a cursory reading of her as a lecherous older woman seducing her footman. While Fielding parodies amatory fiction's language in describing Lady Booby's experience with frustrated desire, her private processing of her passions, shared by a public morality, reveals a verisimilitude of feeling and thinking.

Lady Booby's internal and external speech takes meaning and shape in the historical moment of prescriptive elite English femininity and desire of the time. The coexistence of her utterance within other expressive planes of contradicting belief systems of the medical embodied self and the autonomous Enlightenment being gives bodily form to the dialogic threads in the novel. In *Shamela*, the parody of the aristocratic rake preying on the guileless servant maid mocks the bourgeois values of Puritan sexuality. However, the comic gender reversal and failure of the female seducer in *Joseph Andrews* illuminate Fielding's refracted expression regarding systems of natural desire. Libertine women like Lady Booby do not enjoy the same power as their male counterparts, and as women, they do not pose the same threat of sexual violence. Positioned against higher standards of virtuous behavior than their male peers, these women epitomize monstrous desire. Tiffany Potter observes that Georgian female libertines, with the "freedom and the tools of self determination" unavailable during the Restoration, "concurrently empower and challenge the general qualities of libertinism."[15] Representations of the female libertine's sexuality express a singular and independent sexual desire that depends on popular models of sexuality to resist them. Potter argues that the libertine woman "rejects the assumption of feminine sexual powerlessness, and as a result is one of the few who achieves her status at least partly of her ability to transcend mundane expectations of virtue and culturally prescriptive femininity."[16] Yet, medical and cultural models of the female body's frailty, and how women have internalized these models to understand passion, undercut this capacity to completely move beyond these expectations. And, given how women's sexual excitability is a general factor in discourses of hysteria, especially framed as a way to comprehend women's resistance to a quiet, chaste domesticity, the female libertine's capacity to exercise self-determination is limited.

Samuel Johnson claimed that Fielding produced "characters of nature," characters determined by their manners and discourses.[17] Lady Booby's character is no exception, as readers understand her character patterned by the archetype of a genteel woman of leisure driven by her emotional frailty and excess. While the English physician Thomas Sydenham claims that all women, except for those in the laboring classes who "work and fare hardly," will suffer from hysteria at some point in their lives, the more refined and fragile nervous systems of elite women like Lady Booby put them especially at risk, for it was those "of the liveliest and quickest natural Parts, whose Faculties are the most bright and spiritual, whose Genius is most keen and penetrating, and particularly where there is the most delicate Sensation and Taste" who were predisposed to the disorder.[18] Sydenham gives hysteria's "efficient, internal, and immediate causes" as a "disorder (ataxy) of the animal spirits."[19] This disorder, then, is a physical phenomenon stemming from the nervous fluids' weakened state, which throws the spirits into disarray at the slightest stimulus. Hysteria's source lay in the nervous fluids' structure responsible for muscular movement and the passions. Since hysteria is characterized by fits, or muscular contractions, and disturbances of the passions, with the animal spirits determining muscular movements and the passions, Sydenham concludes that "the disturbance and inconsistency of both the mind and the body" in hysteria stem from a physical difference in the microstructures of the animal spirits.[20] Hence, Sydenham implies that the naturally loose fibers of women's nerves render women more susceptible to the disease. And, comparing hypochondria and hysteria in 1726, the English physician Richard Blackmore attributes hysteric fits' intensity to women's physical constitutions: "the convulsive Disorders and Agitations in the various Parts of the Body, as well as the Confusion and Dissipation of the animal Spirits, are more conspicuous and violent in the Female Sex, than in Men; the reason of which is, a more volatile, dissipable, and weak Constitution of the Spirits, and a more soft, tender, and delicate Texture of the Nerves [among women]."[21] The language used here to describe a woman's experience of passion through the animal spirits—"disturbance," "disorder," "violent"—gestures to a dangerous pathology that calls for the oppressive cultural and medical policing of her body and her self.

In this way, the terms in which medical knowledge of hysteria is understood in the eighteenth century mediates sex roles and gender difference. Ludmilla Jordanova observes that "scientific and medical ideas can be understood as mediations," "that they speak to and contain implications about matters beyond their explicit content."[22] The naturalization of gender difference reinforced by medical knowledge is clear in the ways laypeople imagined how women's bodies worked. Differences of animal spirits' mechanics between men and women, in particular, undergirded explanations of the gendered experience of passion. Haywood herself in *The Female Spectator* refers to the animal spirits to theorize a distinctly female way of processing ideas and thoughts: "The Vivacity of our Ideas, the Quickness of our Apprehensions . . . seem to me to proceed from a greater Redundance of the animal Spirits; and if they sometimes appear too confus'd and hurried, as it were, together, it is but like a Crowd of Mob round the Stage of a Mountebank, where all endeavouring to be foremost, obstruct the Passage of each other."[23] Haywood offers a physiological explanation for the woman's disorderly mind, similar to how one characterizes a hysteric woman's thoughts and actions as "too confus'd and hurried." Haywood's fiction is deeply interested in women's social and medical subjectivity and how the intersections of these two discourses impact how women experience the progress of their passions. While women's bodies and minds were more impressionable than men's in their experience of love, women were also acutely aware of the turbulence in their bodies and possessed enough reason to be cognizant of the hazards in plunging themselves recklessly to fulfill their desires. Lady Booby's private soliloquies dramatize this conflict, demonstrating her emotional intelligence's depth and range.

If a female character's bodily makeup ultimately sets her up for emotional and physical crisis, it would be unsurprising for the author to turn to the amatory form as a means of articulating this crisis. While Fielding parodies the language familiar to Haywood's readers for comic effect—he did satirize her as "Mrs. Novel" in *The Author's Farce* (1730)—amatory language also most authentically represents plots of feeling, the personal emotional experiences of characters, with authorial commentary that analyzes and interprets outcomes from those feelings.[24] In parody, Fielding evokes a variety of points of view, what William Epson called its "double irony": This style encompasses two perspectives but fully supporting neither.[25] And in presenting a character as a female libertine, Fielding illustrates how women experience and process the passions differently from men and how women navigate their worlds as social and scientific subjects.

From the axis of sexual agency and power, female libertines do not wield the same degree of autonomy and dominance as their male counterparts, as dramatized in Lady Booby's failed seduction of Joseph. She coyly asks Joseph, "Would you be contented with a Kiss? Would not your Inclinations be all on fire rather by such a Favour?" "Madam," answers Joseph, "if they were, I hope I should be able to controll them, without suffering them to get the better of my Virtue."[26] Vexed, she rebukes him: "Your Virtue! Have you the Assurance to pretend, that when a Lady demeans herself to throw aside the Rules of Decency, in order to honour you with the highest Favour in her Power, your Virtue should resist Inclination? That when she had conquer'd her own Virtue, she should find an *Obstruction* in yours?" (35). The word "conquer" appears often in medical treatises on the passions to describe the action of overcoming or defeating the impulse to surrender to a self-destructive desire. For example, James Mackenzie asserts in *The History of Health* (1758), "He who seriously resolves to preserve his health, must previously learn to conquer his passions, and to keep them in absolute subjection to reason."[27] (Mackenzie uses the masculine pronoun, but the general advice is for both sexes.)

Passion and reason's binary and hierarchical relationship is explained in military and, by extension, gendered metaphors, with reason as conqueror (imagined as male) and passion as the conquered subject (imagined as female). This power dynamic of conquest plays out often in Haywood's works; Haywood's Fantomina, placing herself in a position of subjection, calls Beauplaisir "all-conquering."[28] While Ronald Paulson imagines the confrontation between Lady Booby and Joseph as an illustration of her "self-delusion, revealing an unhappy, misguided woman who rationalizes her petty affair into a great, theatrical Didoesque love," her outburst reveals more than the idiosyncrasies of a lovelorn subject.[29] In double-voiced discourse, her speech expresses her character's direct intent—to articulate the insult and unexpected rejection—and Fielding's ironic purpose. The reference to herself in the third person, "a Lady," moves the statement from the specific, individual experience to the universal realities of the women she represents. Lady Booby's ironic use of "conquer" does not imply sexual self-restraint, as Mackenzie's use of the word does; rather, by "throwing aside rules of decency," rules requiring female sexual governance, she overthrows or "conquers" the patriarchal regime that determines the laws of female conduct to open a space in which she can position herself to be subjected, or conquered, by her footman.

Both Fielding and Haywood (especially in Haywood's 1748 novel *Life's Progress through the Passions; or, The Adventures of Natura*) explicitly committed to realism and moral seriousness in their novels, and both dramatize women's failure in managing their passions. In *Joseph Andrews*, Lady Booby, "enraged at her disappointment" (29) in Joseph's refusal to join her "naked in Bed" (25), struggles with her decision to dismiss Joseph, "after much tossing and turning her Bed, and many Soliloquies" (30). Before making her final decision, she resolves to "examine him" after "the little God *Cupid*, fearing he had not yet done the Lady's Business, took a fresh Arrow with the sharpest Point in his Quiver, and shot it directly into her Heart: in other plainer Language, the Lady's Passion got the better of her Reason" (31). Employing amatory language in Cupid as metaphor for comic effect, Fielding draws Lady Booby's body as an entity that external agents acted on (and the arrow's phallic overtones can hardly be missed). And with passion overcoming reason, the two are illustrated as opposing forces. Lady Booby's experience here dramatizes the apparent conflict between rationality and emotion, but the convergence of the cultural, psychological, and historical contingencies presents a more complicated view.[30] To show this complication further, after Joseph's departure, she "burst[s] forth" the following reflection: "Whither doth this violent Passion hurry us? What Meannesses do we submit to from its impulse? Wisely we resist its first and least Approaches; for it is then only we can assure ourselves the Victory. No woman could ever safely say, so far only will I go" (36). Lady Booby's attribution of her weakness in character to her body's essential frailty echoes Blackmore's language describing hysteria symptoms as violent and unique to women's physical constitutions. The nature of women's animal spirits as liable to rapid, unpredictable change coursing through fragile nerves renders her doubly subservient to her passions, especially when we consider the mechanics of the passions conceived by medical thinkers and philosophers such as Thomas Willis on the anatomy of the brain and the nervous system and by John Locke on epistemology.[31] The mechanics of the passions imply that the individual is being acted on instead of operating independently, as Stephen Ahern notes: "Such a model of embodied being complicates the picture of the individual as autonomous and self-determining that has long been seen as a legacy of the Enlightenment."[32] What is more, many eighteenth-century figures have written on their intensities of feeling to "generate a kind of existential disorientation that results from a feeling of lack of control over self."[33] This "existential disorientation" is mediated through the romance as a "mode of representation" in its rhetorical and emotional excess of the pining lover, previously seen in narratives of amorous intrigue of the 1680s to the 1720s.[34] Lady Booby processes the passions' violence into voluntary abjection for sexual union and, thus, fulfillment. Within the amatory framework, the desiring subject positions herself in the submissive role for her desire to be sated. Ahern explains the emotional contradiction in the romance mode's "love theory": "The paradox of this ideal of romantic love is that although it promises a transcendent 'transport' of erotic communion, the ecstatic mingling of the souls and the bodies of lovers destined for one another, there is an implicit violence in its terms and assumptions."[35] The loss of self-possession is requisite for the state of exquisite sexual feeling. The violence felt through the passions is expressed by the desire for violence on the self.

Drawing from Haywood's lexicon and style of expressing emotional struggle works toward Fielding's comic effect—diluting the strength of Lady Booby's sexual threat as ridiculous—but the style of these expressions also functions as a vehicle that acknowledges woman as the bodily theater in which the philosophical debates of the relationship of emotion and reason are staged. Haywood's readers will find this conflict between reason and passion, between duty and desire, as a familiar "feature of aesthetic excess" in her novels.[36] Mary Anne Schofield describes Haywood's narratives to reflect on the prevailing sex-gender hierarchies, with the masculine as the position of power that both idealized and infantilized the feminine. Dramatizing the path to self-realization, heroines struggle against contradictory bourgeois expectations for women: "Haywood's heroines give vicarious expression to both the exterior and interior life of eighteenth-century women. Haywood's typical heroine presents a docile, subdued face to society but reveals a shockingly turbulent, aggressive interior to those who probe beneath her facade."[37] Ahern builds on Schofield's study, noting that "the main contradiction Haywood explores plays out as a conflict between, on the one hand, sexual desire and duty to self (in the drive to self-fulfillment), and on the other, duty to the larger community (in the drive to conform to expectation by satisfying only those desires that are socially sanctioned)."[38] Haywood's amatory novels centralize the female characters' struggles between their duty to self and community. This conflict is not the major thematic concern in *Joseph Andrews* or *Tom Jones*, but Fielding addresses the singular experience of the desiring woman through Lady Booby in explicitly sexual terms outside the marriage model. Fanny desires and loves Joseph, and Sophia desires and loves Tom, but these couplings orient toward marriage to consummate and legitimize their desire in adherence to the comic mode's happy ending. Through Fanny and Sophia, Fielding identifies regulated female desire as a primary moral source in an ordered society. Therefore, moral anxiety shades Lady Booby's voluntary abjection in her drive to self-fulfillment.

Libertine women, through their resistance to the hegemonic sphere of influence, essentially reinforce the imposed worldview that justifies and naturalizes the social status quo. Their attempt to exercise social and sexual self-determination by giving in to their passions, a transgression against prescriptive femininity, gives credence to the idea that women's bodies were more likely to be sexually stimulated from inadequate biological adaptive mechanisms to regulate their passions. Excitability, particularly sexual excitability, persists in discourses of hysteria. This belief can be traced as far back as Galen, who maintained that sex deprivation could lead to hysteria.[39] The Scottish physician William Cullen claimed that hysteria "occurs especially in females who are liable to nymphomania," including the classification *Hysterica libidonosa* for such a woman in his writings.[40] Some physicians, like William Harvey, adopted the contrary view, that marriage (with its socially sanctioned conjugal benefits) would cure the hysterical female.[41] The "violent passion" that provides the impetus for sexual excitability that women experienced, as Lady Booby declares here, distinguishes their inferior difference from their male counterparts. Male libertines, even in their sexual appetite's excess, own themselves from the bodily superiority attributed to male bodies.

Physicians delineated bodies' physiological hierarchy even at the vascular level. Though physicians diagnosed men with hysterical symptoms (usually identified as hypochondria), hysteria was generally understood as a common female disease that the woman's biological makeup caused. The professor of medicine Herman Boerhaave theorized that the hydraulic model of the female body's vascular system works against her healthiness. Boerhaave proposed that women's "Fibres" are "generally lax and loose," compared with "the solid Parts" of adult males and laborers.[42] English physician John Freind confirms Boerhaave's opinion, citing women's weakness arising from smaller holes in the blood vessels: "Orifices of the vessels be much smaller in Women than in Men (which perhaps is not repugnant to Reason, because both their Frame is more finely and delicately put together, and their Bulk always more contracted)."[43] The difference in women's vascular structure from men's means, then, a concomitant difference in how women and men experience their passions. Women's "lax and loose" "fibres" render them unable to develop healthy adaptive mechanisms, resulting in a state of "existential disorientation." Taken as a whole, medical discourse contradicts the Enlightenment promise of the autonomous and self-determining being, at least for women. Nerve theory's language here makes plain that this promise is reserved only for men with the "solid parts" necessary to regulate their passions. Women's desires code differently in a culture that identifies them as the primary moral source, and therefore, women's physiological experiences of their passions can never operate outside cultural or ethical registers. The way that women view their own physical responses is always mediated by the cultural expectations for restraint, even as medical discourse directly conflicts this physiological inability for women to regulate their emotional excess. In representing Lady Booby's inner struggle that considers social duty in her drive to sexual self-fulfillment, Fielding expresses an ambivalence in the strict conflation of sexual desire and moral sensibility.

Fielding further demonstrates this inner discord—practicing restraint and indulging in pleasure—in the realm of dreams. If women's bodies are subject to arousing stimuli, then that stimuli's removal would give them a measure of relief. In that same line of logic, the stimuli's return would then revive familiar emotional turbulence. Lady Booby's "second Appearance . . . on the Stage" confirms the indelible impression of desire and the violence that this unfulfilled desire wreaks on her mind and body. Fielding returns to amatory language in the metaphor of Cupid to describe her experience: "the Arrow had pierced deeper than she imagined; nor was the wound so easily cured. The Removal of the Object soon cooled her Rage, but it had a different Effect on her Love; that departed with his Person; but this remained lurking in her mind with his Image" (242). Fielding merges amatory and medical language in the "wound" metaphor; her desire for Joseph is represented as a chronic injury from which she continues to suffer. So deep is the "wound" that it manifests as nightmares and fantasies: "Restless, interrupted slumbers, and confused horrible dreams were her portion the first night. In the morning, fancy painted her a more delicious scene; but to delude, not delight her: for before she could reach the promised happiness, it vanished, and left her to curse, not bless the vision" (242). Fielding articulates Lady Booby's experience of unfulfilled desire through amatory language, but within the framework of hysteria. She feels exquisite pleasure in the "delicious scene" of illusion in her dreams, only to "curse" it when she discovers her reality. Nightmares and "disturbances of the imagination," Heather Meek observes, were common symptoms of hysteria written in medical texts.[44] The physician Robert Whytt reported "disturbed sleep, frightful dreams, [and] the night-mare" in cases of hysteric patients.[45] Haywood theorizes how these manifestations of unfulfilled desire work in her novels, as Aleksondra Hultquist observes: "Haywood's work develops an ethics of passionate experience: her prose effectively forms a vocabulary for the passions, demonstrates their significance in the experience of the fictional characters, and analyses the outcomes through authorial commentary."[46] For example, in *Love in Excess* (1719–1720), Haywood outlines how women's prohibited desires can manifest in vividly sensual dreams, even if the woman practices virtuous composure in her waking hours: "But whatever Dominion, Honour and Virtue may have over our waking Thoughts, 'tis certain that they fly from the clos'd Eyes, our Passions then exert their forceful Power, and that which is most Predominant in the Soul, agitates the Fancy, and brings even Things impossible to pass: Desire, with watchful Diligence repell'd, returns with greater Violence in unguarded Sleep, and overthrows the vain Efforts of Day."[47] Again, reason and passion present as entities waging war on the battlegrounds of the woman's body. A woman's effort to repress or deny desire is an unavailing exercise, as her body's vascular mechanics work against her. In Haywood's rendering, this repression is worse since desire "returns with greater Violence." Returning to Fielding's personification of desire that opened this chapter, the nightmare is the "window" in which "Nature" creeps through.

In creating a character dominated by her emotional life, Fielding follows Haywood's philosophical view that the best approach to ordering the passions is to counterbalance with another kind of passion, not with reason. Fielding traces Lady Booby's passions from Joseph's reappearance, representing the range of feelings similar to Haywood's system of understanding the progress of passion. He details how her desire runs its violent course through her body and mind, and ultimately, this leads her to seek relief: "Reflection then hurried her farther, and told her she must see this beautiful Youth no more, nay, suggested to her, that she herself had dismissed him for no other Fault, than probably that of too violent an Awe and Respect for herself. . . . She then blamed, she cursed the hasty Rashness of her Temper; her Fury was vented all on herself, and Joseph appeared innocent in her Eyes. Her Passion at length grew so violent that it forced on her seeking Relief" (242). Her passion's violence forcing her to seek relief implies her loss of bodily control. To free herself from distress, her passions must be given vent. Frustrated, she turns the blame inward to herself, to impulsively acting on her anger. But then, she finds a counterbalance to her passion: "Prid forbad that, Pride which soon drove all softer Passions from her Soul, and represented to her the Meanness of him she was fond of" (242). Emotional fickleness and inconstancy, in the same way Lady Booby demonstrates here, have been determined by physicians as inherent symptoms of hysteria. Richard Blackmore writes that hysteria "embroils" the mind's "Government and Operations [from] whence proceed Diffidence, Suspicion, Inconstancy, Timidity, Irresolution, Change of Temper, Judgment and Resolution; as likewise excessive Gaiety of Temper, or the contrary Extreme."[48] Physicians simply reduce women's wildly vacillating emotional states to their disordered bodies as the root of the problem. However, Lady Booby's mental and emotional anguish is a *reflection* of her inner turmoil in choosing love over duty and reputation, not necessarily from some inherent biological cause.

Distressing passion can be neutralized by another kind of feeling, a common phenomenon that Hultquist notes in Haywood's understanding of the passions: "Rather than passions being controlled through careful reason, stoicism, or prayer, as they had been in past configurations, Haywood remarks upon the ways in which the passions themselves counterbalance and create a self."[49] The reader is taken through the spectrum of intense feeling that Lady Booby experiences as she reflects on her disappointed lust for Joseph: fury, contempt, disdain, hatred, pleasure:

> That thought soon began to obscure his beauties; contempt succeeded next, and then disdain, which presently introduced her hatred of the creature who had given her so much uneasiness. These enemies of Joseph had no sooner taken possession of her mind, than they insinuated to her a thousand things in his disfavor. . . . Revenge came now to her assistance; and she considered her dismission of him stript, and without a character, with the utmost pleasure. She rioted in the several kinds of misery, which her imagination suggested to her, might be his fate; and with a smile composed anger, mirth, and scorn, viewed him in the rags in which her fancy had drest him. (243)

Through her imagination, Lady Booby takes herself from abject vulnerability to gratifying vengeance. In earlier scenes, reason and passion battled in a positive/negative continuum, but later, this system of emotion views passionate traits as compensating each other.[50] Later, Lady Booby reflects on Mrs. Slipslop's comically malapropistic suggestion to follow her desire, since her "Ladyship hath no Parents to tutelar your Infections," and Joseph, discovered later as Pamela's brother, is "as good a Gentleman as any in the country" (287). In anguished soliloquy, Lady Booby considers the possibility of settling with Joseph, despite the public scandal it would cause ("I can retire from them; retire with one in whom I propose more Happiness than the World without him can give me!"), deprecates her feelings ("Ha! And do I doat thus on a Footman? I despise, I detest my passion."), weighs his virtues ("Is he not generous, gentle, kind?"), condemns his love for Fanny ("Kind to whom? To the meanest Wretch, a Creature below my Consideration."), and finally decides to scorn him ("No, I will tear his Image from my Bosom, tread on him, spurn him.") (288). Though Lady Booby attributes the "Aids of Reason" in her choice not to "sacrifice . . . Reputation . . . Character . . . Rank in Life, to the Indulgence of a mean and vile Appetite," she thanks her "Pride" for having "perfectly conquered this unworthy Passion" (288). Motivations come from the passions; thus, action results from the passions, not reason.

And it is the progress of Lady Booby's passions that drives her character and the novel's plot. Her attempts to thwart Fanny and Joseph's wedding set the novel's course into its near-incest drama, then into its final resolution, in which the power balance is restored through the reaffirmation of the genteel and patriarchal Booby and Wilson families. This closing is in keeping with the structural plot of the comic novel, in which domestic harmony is reestablished, with the material futures of deserving characters secured. And perhaps, in an act of compassion, Fielding gives Lady Booby a version of a happy ending: "she returned to London in a few days, where a young Captain of Dragoons, together with eternal Parties at Cards, soon obliterated the Memory of Joseph" (303). She is able to vent her passions with another young man, and the wound created by the memory of her unrequited love for Joseph has scarred over.

Lady Booby, as Potter rightly claims, reflects and evaluates her emotional and bodily responses more than any other figure in the novel.[51] While Paul Baines calls her a "wicked stepmother" and "breaker of all the rules of rank, age, and gender," he concedes that Lady Booby offers more depth and emotional range than the novel's heroine, Fanny: "Much of what might be termed the internal psychological processing of the novel is concentrated on Lady Booby's tormented self-deceptions and internal vacillations, on which Fielding expends considerable energy, bordering on a kind of sympathy."[52] So why would Fielding spend all this energy on a single character's interior and emotional life? On this score, I argue that while Fielding is interested in public performance in authenticity of representation and character as a satirist, Lady Booby's characterization demonstrates how feeling drives plot. Lady Booby's displays of excess are not tangential qualities in drawing a character for satiric effect; rather, her emotional excess is a central element in the narrative. And unlike Mrs. Slipslop's grotesque, carnal aggression, Lady Booby's desires are framed as scenes of suffering, progressing through an emotional range that delivers moments of pathos. Additionally, the verisimilitude of her inner life articulates and confirms hysteria as a cultural metaphor that defends the medical views of women's bodies as inherently pathological in the resistance against the ideal of passive feminine chastity. Paradoxically, Fielding parodies the rhetoric of amatory fiction's emotional excess only to represent the emotional lives of desiring women in an authentic and honest way. As a woman who questions the cultural mores of her time, who seriously considers subverting traditional limitations for the sake of feminine self-determination, who admits and acts on her desire, Lady Booby, in my estimation, is far from a simple caricature of a lovesick villainess.

## HYSTERICAL LETTERS OF THE LIBERTINE SINGLE WOMAN

Compared to Lady Booby, Lady Bellaston's status as a libertine single woman in *Tom Jones* enacts an even more subversive expression of female desire, as she does not share the same degree of concern over social duty as Lady Booby does as a feature of her aesthetic excess. Not only does Lady Bellaston openly embrace her identity as a single woman who enjoys sexual liaisons (a status ostensibly dangerous to herself, as she is without the protection of a male head) and who "often ridiculed romantic love" (607), but she is also ideologically opposed to the institution of marriage. She proclaims that she will protect women who suffer under the tyranny of their fathers or husbands: "I shall ever esteem it the cause of my sex to rescue any woman who is so unfortunate to be under their power" (609). After fleeing from her father's attempt to force her into marriage with the odious Blifil, Sophia Western finds refuge in her cousin Lady Bellaston's London residence: "[Lady Bellaston] highly applauded [Sophia's] sense and resolution; and after expressing the highest satisfaction in the opinion which Sophia had declared she entertained of her ladyship, by chusing her house for an asylum, she promised her all the protection which it was in her power to give" (538). The individual autonomy and shifting power that interest Lady Bellaston, evidenced by her belief in absolute sexual freedom and her fascination with disguise, are major features of libertinism.[53] Potter writes, "[Lady Bellaston] challenges social norms not only in her open sexuality, but also in her independent repudiation of the concept of marriage as an institution repressive to women, her use of the libertine topoi of the masquerade and disguise as tools of her liberty, and her effective manipulations and deceptions of others in pursuit of power and her other desires."[54] By all accounts, the libertinism of Lady Bellaston, as an economically independent woman who enjoys sex outside of marriage and who advocates the same pleasures and freedoms for other women, exudes a refreshing, insurrectionary protofeminist energy that threatens to upend the value of male authority and the myths of domesticity in the novel. But in adherence to the comic tradition, Lady Bellaston's hysterical excesses and gender transgressions are ultimately contained in the return to domestic harmony by the novel's end. Her assertions of sexual agency briefly create the tension to drive the narrative toward its resolution and serve as the novel's explicit satirical aims in the importance of domestic and social order.

Despite Lady Bellaston's proclaimed support for victimized women, she abandons her homosocial relationship with Sophia for Tom's affections. Later, driven by a burning jealousy, she schemes to destroy their love by attempting to permanently separate them. Lady Bellaston's choice for sexual conquest over homosocial friendship is reminiscent of the libertine character Melantha in Haywood's *Love in Excess* (1719), who has no qualms over betraying her friend Alovisa, the wife of D'elmont: "I care not. . . . I have set my heart on an hours diversion with him, and will not be baulked if the repose of the world, much less that of a jealous, silly wife, depended on it."[55] Lady Bellaston's inexorable desire drives the narrative's plot, her intensities of feeling mediated through the romance mode in her rhetorical and emotional excess as the jilted lover seen in earlier narratives of amatory intrigue. In *Tom Jones*, Fielding turns to the epistolary form—a rhetorical device familiar in amatory fiction—to give insight on how women process their passions in a style that could be categorized as hysterical.

As mentioned earlier in this chapter, practitioners considered women's defiance against prescriptive domesticity as a manifestation of self-inflicted hysteria, a kind of punishment for renegade women who openly displayed their sexuality. Fielding's later iteration of the female libertine in Lady Bellaston, following Lady Booby, figures as a flippant rebel who refuses to submit to the conventional gender hierarchy formalized through the institution of marriage. As an unmarried woman, *by choice*, she will, according to medical practitioners, continue to suffer from hysteria in refusing to accept her place. Single women were particularly at risk of experiencing hysterical symptoms. Richard Mead's *Medical Precepts and Cautions* (1751) begins a section on "the diseases of women" with "those, which are often the consequences of a single life."[56] However, this single, hysterical life implies a chaste one. John Ball strongly prescribes marriage for single women suffering from hysterical symptoms: "If the patient be single and of a proper age, the advice of Hippocrates should be followed, who wisely says, that *a woman's best remedy is to marry, and bear children*."[57] Marital sex will ostensibly alleviate the hysterical symptoms of single women. And yet, Lady Bellaston—and many of the unmarried libertine women in Haywood's novels—enjoys sex acts without a husband. Lady Bellaston's example repudiates the medical principle and reveals that the disciplining mechanism of marriage, not sex, cures hysterical women. Ultimately, marriage's heteronormative and monogamous features regulate desire, a regulation that Lady Bellaston vehemently rejects.

The other aspect of marriage that purportedly cured the hysterical woman was the prospect of becoming pregnant and giving birth. Ancient medical tradition viewed the uterus, also called the "mother," as the seat of hysteria and the root of all female disease. In the "wandering womb" theory, pregnancy anchors the uterus from floating up and suffocating the woman, alleviating her hysterical symptoms for the short term. Framed in this way, pregnancy benefits women and perpetuates the mythology of the joyful (and healthy) domesticity of the mother. Conversely, sex acts outside of reproductive futurity took an immoral dimension in the institutions of both marriage and nation. Haywood's contemporary Daniel Defoe makes this clear in *Conjugal Lewdness; or, Matrimonial Whoredom* (1726): "Matrimony was instituted for the regular Propagation of Kind," and "preposterous" women who choose not to have children "would have the Use of a Man, but would not act the Part of the Woman."[58] Richard Smalbroke, the bishop of St. David's, emphasized the national duty to procreate in his 1728 sermon: "whatever has a direct Tendency to lessen the Number of Subjects, and to weaken or dishonor the Government, or bring it in to Confusion, falls under [the Magistrate's] immediate Cognizance."[59] Women's civic disenfranchisement directly correlated with their role in reproduction. Women's physical frailty necessitated their subordination to men in both their families and the government. Lady Bellaston, however, repudiates subservience to either to maintain complete control over her own wealth and independence. In her ambition to preserve sexual and financial agency, she is cast as a monstrous exploiter of sexual and national politics.

## *Straight Out of Haywood*

Lady Bellaston has been categorized as masculine; as Terry Castle observes, Lady Bellaston usurps masculine privilege by living a "life of sexual self-gratification more properly suited to male libertines."[60] Nightingale assures Tom, "You are not the first young fellow she hath debauched" (718). Framed as another simple gender reversal like Lady Booby, Lady Bellaston becomes the seducer and corrupter of innocent young men. But I think the more fitting and accurate comparison here is not with libertine men (as I have shown earlier that women's emotional processing and understanding of this processing render that as an impossibility) but with libertine women in early amatory fiction. *The Injur'd Husband*'s Baroness de Tortillée, *The Perplex'd Dutchess; or, Treachery Rewarded*'s Gigantilla, and *The Force of Nature; or, The Lucky Disappointment*'s Alantha are all Haywood characters who mimic the vile excesses of libertine men, and all are rejected by Haywood for their unbridled passion destructive to themselves and to the world.[61] The Baroness de Tortillée, in particular, shares the same qualities as Lady Bellaston; through relentless and careful manipulation, and with the help of her lackey Du Lache, the Baroness collects and discards men under the cover of her title, all while assuming a virtuous facade. Andrea Austin notes the "double bind" that women experience in Haywood's novels: "a woman who desires freedom and an equal share of life's entertainments puts herself in serious danger, but a woman who denies herself these things and maintains the character of a 'proper' woman risks giving up all authority over her own life."[62] There is protection in women's passivity, so the libertine woman, as a sexually and socially active person, risks herself and others on whom she will inflict pain and injury in endeavoring control over her own life in the fulfillment of her desires. And if the security of the family and the nation rests on the passivity of its women subjects, active women threaten this balance. Through the moral and medical framing of hysteria, women like Lady Bellaston, who stubbornly reject submission to the conventional gender hierarchy entrenched in the institution of marriage, inflict hysterical symptoms onto themselves. As I explain further in this chapter, these symptoms become legible in the epistolary form and in their intemperate indulgence of vengeance.

## *The Epistolary Form as the Mediator of Emotion*

In *Tom Jones*, Fielding returns to the amatory form as a means of articulating a woman's emotional and physical crisis in processing desire, but with a significant difference: Lady Booby's inner turbulence is mediated through the narrator in a form closer to parody, while Lady Bellaston's emotional spiraling is registered directly in the epistolary form, a genre commonly associated with the feminine. While the reader is given access to Lady Booby's interiority to witness her "Confusion of Spirits," Fielding adopts epistolary narration as an alternative method to convey Lady Bellaston's hysterical mercuriality. Fielding read Richardson's *Clarissa* (1748) while he was composing the latter half of *Tom Jones*, which may explain its comparatively heavier use of letters for storytelling in his novel. In double irony once more, Fielding encompasses both perspectives of mocking the writing-to-the-moment he previously criticized in Richardson's *Pamela*, then admired in *Clarissa*, and acknowledges the authenticity of feeling and immediate temporality delivered through the epistolary mode. Richardson writes in his preface to *Clarissa*, "All the letters are written while the hearts of the writers must be supposed to be wholly engaged in their subjects. . . . So that they abound not only with critical Situations, but with what may be called *instantaneous* Descriptions and Reflections."[63] In contrast to Fielding's contempt with Pamela's insincerity in *Shamela*, he admired the more balanced and human *Clarissa* and was greatly affected by this narrative style in his own reading of the novel and his stylization of *Tom Jones*. In 1748, he wrote a letter of praise to his rival, tracing the registers of emotions he experienced in his reading: "Here my Terror ends and my Grief begins which is the Cause of all my Tumultuous Passions and soon changes into Raptures of Admiration and Astonishment."[64] But unlike Richardson's female characters, who inhabit a narrative world where the Augustan frame of values renders them as quiescent agents, Fielding's Lady Bellaston blurs the boundaries of the relative power of men and women, contravening the common presentation of women as passive victims.

In libertine fashion, Lady Bellaston begins her affair with Tom under her own clandestine terms. The seduction opens at a masquerade, another familiar convention of amatory fiction and befitting her character as a libertine woman. Ros Ballaster suggests that the masquerade in Haywood's early works empowered women characters, "making [them] a weaver and dilator of [their] own amatory plot. . . . The masquerade functions as a site in which gender inversion and amatory activity is licensed under the sanction of organised 'secrecy.'"[65] Lady Bellaston then begins her covert campaign to seduce Tom by delivering a bundle with a domino, a mask, a masquerade ticket, and a mystery billet from "the queen of the fairies" (619). Desperately hoping that this invitation came from Mrs. Fitzpatrick, whom Tom imagines as an ally for helping him find Sophia, he attends the masquerade with Nightingale. He encounters a woman with a domino mask whom he mistakenly believes is Mrs. Fitzpatrick, and both engage in a flirtatious exchange. The woman expresses her boredom at the masquerade, and Tom attends her to her lodgings in secret, where he discovers that the masked woman is Lady Bellaston. Terry Castle claims that masquerades were "equated with the sexual act itself; the metonymic relation between masquerades and sex becomes a metaphoric one."[66]

The masquerade seduction directed by Lady Bellaston is consummated (as it is implied offstage in the narration), and afterward, she sets the terms for their subsequent liaisons. Through her exploitation of Tom's poverty, Lady Bellaston maintains control over the sexual and power dynamic between them. Torn between his devotion to Sophia and his sexual obligations to Lady Bellaston, Tom "knew the tacit consideration upon which all her favours were conferred; and as his necessity obliged him to accept them, so his honour, he concluded, forced him to pay the price" (634). Lady Bellaston's "violent fondness" for her lover, carried out in secrecy, becomes public through Tom's upgraded appearance: "by her means he was now become one of the best-dressed men about town, . . . raised to a state of affluence beyond what he had ever known" (633). The commentary regarding Lady Bellaston's passions for Tom remains secondary, and readers can only glean from the narrator's descriptions of their meetings (with the prurient or amorous material omitted out of propriety) and Tom's appearance and reflections.

However, Lady Bellaston's intensities of feeling for Tom become explicit once she suspects him of carrying on a secret affair with Sophia. Lady Bellaston had arranged an evening with Tom at her lodgings, sending Sophia away to a play for that time. By chance, Lady Bellaston is delayed from her dinner, and Sophia returns early. In a tense episode, each character denies the truth of each other's acquaintance, and Tom imagines himself preserved. Almost immediately upon his arrival home, he receives a series of angry letters from Lady Bellaston that dramatize her passions and jealousy. The content and style of these letters could be characterized as hysteric; the somatic symptoms of hysteria were usually accompanied by psychological or emotional symptoms such as capriciousness, irritability, manic mood swings, periods of delirious ravings or unintelligible talk, and paranoia.[67] Blackmore describes hysterical patients as experiencing "Fluctuation of Judgement, and swift Turns in forming and reversing Opinions and Resolutions, . . . Absence of Mind, want of self-determining Power, Inattention, Incogitancy, Diffidence, Suspicion, and an Aptness to take well-meant Things amiss."[68] The physician Nicholas Robinson notes the extreme swings of the hysterical lover: As hysterics are "wavering and unsteady in their Judgments, neither do they observe a Rectitude in any one Action of Life: Now they love a Person to Excess, presently after they hate him in the other Extreme; anon they resolve to do such an Action, a Moment after they alter their purpose, and take directly contrary Measures."[69]

Lady Bellaston's first letter is a medley of self-rebuke for loving Tom, whom she believes is besotted with "an idiot," paranoia ("Was this scheme laid between you"), and menace ("remember, I can detest as violently as I have loved"; 651). In Haywood's *Life's Progress through the Passions: or, the Adventures of Natura* (1748), anger is "the most violent emotions of the soul" borne from pride; "it is by the dictates of this pernicious passion we are inflamed with wrath, and wild ambition,—instigated to covetousness,—to envy,—to revenge, and in fine, to stop at nothing which tends to self gratification, to be our desires of what kind soever."[70] For men, reason comes with age to regulate anger: "whereas wrath diminishes as our reason increases, and seems intirely evaporated after the heat of youth is over: when a man therefore has divested himself of the one, no tokens are left to distinguish the other" (18). Haywood refers to "we," the general public, in her explanation of the workings of pride and its secondary passions, but she identifies only men as developing the capacity for reason to counterbalance this passion as they age. This is not to say that Haywood is implying that women lack the capacity to use reason or to regulate their emotions; rather, as illustrated in many of her early amatory narratives, women engaging in the fantasy of rebellion and liberation ultimately realize the limitations of female ambition. It is during these moments when the limitations are felt as real, the fantasy dissolves, and the woman's emotional experiences are registered as hysterical.

The epistolary form uniquely highlights Enlightenment binaries of gender embodiment, with the letter exposing the tension between the private and the public at the risk of the letter writer. "The letter-narrative," according to Elizabeth Cook, makes visible the "tension" between private gendered subjectivity and a public identity, for it "exposes the private body to publication."[71] Moreover, while letters were associated with spontaneity of feeling, women still had to cope with censoring the letter's material so as not to transgress decorum. Writing on letters and censorship in the period, Barbara Zaczek makes clear that the disciplining of women's desires occurred within their bodies and by their pens.[72] Thus, Lady Bellaston's sexual excesses and futile attempts to restrain those excesses also translate into her epistolary excesses, an example of how print renders her hysterical body more visible, in the same ways Shamela's and Win's letters do.

The rapidly vacillating intensities of feeling in Lady Bellaston's scrawls align with the medical narrative of women's gender frailty as embodied beings. Her epistolary style recalls the hyperbolic constructions of earlier amatory narratives, specifically her use of fragmented speech, with broken phrases in between typographical marks of interruption, such as dashes. These dashes convey a hysterical hurriedness in the composition, as if searching for language in the text itself: "For though [Sophia] understood not a word of what passed between us, yet she had the skill, the assurance, the—what shall I call it?—to deny to my face that she knows you" (651). These formal techniques, Ahern notes, "work to generate a sense of heightened drama" and "constitute the formal apparatus of a narrative mode that proceeds from the fundamental assumption that the reader shares an intense interest in the minute changes that occur in a lover's emotional and psychophysiological registers."[73] And, indeed, tension has been building from the last scene, with the characters in a love triangle. Though each believed they had escaped with their secrets preserved, the dangerous and volatile passion of one simmers, threatening to explode. What is more, the belief that women's nerves are liable to swift and mercurial change portend a catastrophic event, as Lady Bellaston's emotions veer outside of her control. Through the letter's composition, the reader is kept in suspense of what could possibly happen next.

Fielding also uses another hyperbolic construction in amatory fiction, the repetition of sentence structure, particularly through the postscript. Attempting to neutralize the situation, Lady Bellaston sends another letter explicitly attributing the "rather too warm" (717) note to the disorder of her animal spirits. However, the subsequent set of correspondence betrays her excess in hysteric utterances. The three lines of postscripts following the second letter emphasize her impatience and urgency: "P.S. I have ordered to be at home to none but yourself. P.S. Mr Jones will imagine I shall assist him in his defence; for I believe he cannot desire to impose on me more than I desire to impose on myself. P.S. Come immediately" (651). Richard Terry asserts in his study on the postscript in eighteenth-century literature that this epistolary device tends to "flourish most in amorous correspondence, as especially facilitating secret affairs or elopements, and as belonging to an epistolary territory over which women were the acknowledged rulers."[74] Postscripts also tend to be a sign of "amorous distraction," more "emotionally abandoned": "Postscript . . . marks the boundary between reason and unreason, between self-control and emotional abandonment. The heart spills out from its confines at the same time as the letter spills out beyond its formal close."[75] Again, existential disorientation is mediated through amatory language, even at the textual level of letters. The multiple postscripts materialize the mood swings and paranoia of the hysterical woman's body. Lady Bellaston's ungovernable emotions, more than anything else—her interactions with others, her reflections mediated by the narrator—are authentically and directly represented for the reader through the epistolary form.

Lady Bellaston's passions as registered in her writing are shortly confirmed through her body by the external observer. The tempo of time during this episode is lightning quick, the demonstrations of intense feeling occurring in rapid succession. Immediately after Tom reads her second letter, she enters Tom's lodgings "very disordered in her dress" and "very discomposed in her looks" (651). Ahern has noted the repetition of "silent displays of emotional excess" in Haywood's characters: "Frozen in the moment of overwhelming emotion, they form *tableaux vivants* that testify with extravagant gesture to the intensity of the present experience."[76] After a pause, Lady Bellaston explains herself to Tom, saying, "You see, sir, when women have gone one length too far, they will stop at none. If any person would have sworn this to me a week ago, I would not have believed it of myself" (652). Like Lady Booby, she speaks for all women, but with a difference: Once a transgression has been made, women, having given in to their excesses, become indefatigable in fulfilling their desires. Lady Bellaston's existential disorientation—"I would not have believed it myself"—splits her consciousness and self in two, existing in both the past and the present: The past self disbelieves the actions of the present self at the present time. The present desiring self, with the past self as a censorious presence, a kind of superego, is positioned for violence in voluntary abjection for sexual union. Lady Bellaston's awareness of her own humiliation stands as an example of how women knowingly inflict hysterical symptoms on themselves. For eighteenth-century medical practitioners, she deserves her suffering and abjection; by flaunting her sexuality and indulging in socially unsanctioned desire, she is weakening her already-fragile nerves. The woman's "more volatile, dissipable, and weak Constitution of the Spirits," according to Blackmore, causes her to experience passion in "more conspicuous and violent" ways. And genteel women like Lady Bellaston, whose nervous systems render them more vulnerable to hysterical symptoms, must carefully regulate their behavior to protect themselves from psychosomatic suffering. Her failure to do so, as she dives headfirst into her possessive infatuation with Tom, operates as a caution and affirmation of the harm that libertine women bring onto themselves. Without the same regulatory systems of the "solid" bodies of men, female libertines are physically and emotionally incapable of indulging in the same freedoms.

Fielding uses the epistolary form most energetically in a single chapter, aptly titled "Containing love-letters of several sorts" (717). In a similar response in discovering Sophia and Tom together, Lady Bellaston demands an explanation for Sophia's maidservant Honour's appearance, sending three notes commanding Tom's immediate presence at her side. She explains her existential disorientation as being "under some strange infatuation" (717). Her emotional volatility has deepened: "I cannot keep my resolutions a moment" (717). The textual style of the letters reflects her emotional state of passionate excess: dashes, incomplete thoughts, and repetition. "Come to me, therefore, the moment you receive this. . . . Betrayed to—I will think no more.—Come to me directly. . . . Come to me presently." She understands the risks of writing these letters in her state: This is "the third letter [she has] writ, the two former are burnt." With this letter, she is "almost inclined to burn this too," admitting that she wishes she could "preserve [her] senses" (717). Lady Bellaston reproduces the immediacy of her body's internal struggle between passion and reason (or her "senses"), and both Tom and the reader can trace the instantaneous changes in the lover's emotional registers. While she notes that she should check her feelings and exercise restraint, she ultimately leans into her pursuit of fulfilling her desire with reckless abandon. Two shorter billets follow, one with an ultimatum ("If you ever expect to be forgiven, or even suffered within my doors, come to me this instant"), the other with more consideration ("I now find you was not at home when my notes came. . . . The moment you receive this let me see you. . . . Sure nothing can detain you long" (717). Considering the breadth of time covered in the novel, Lady Bellaston's hysterical unraveling occurs in shortly spaced bursts of intensity in her letters. In every other public appearance, she exercises a cold, aloof, and imperial restraint. Fielding carves out a space in the narrative to provide insight into her emotional processing, showing the levels of desperation she has reached, perhaps helping the audience understand the cruel injuries she attempts to inflict later on Sophia and Tom. Without giving us access into her interiority, Fielding would erase her humanity, rendering her as a flat, lovesick villainess.

### *Vengeance as Cure*

The common cure for hysteria, as many practitioners have suggested, was sexual intercourse for the married patient or marriage for the single woman. As a libertine woman, Lady Bellaston enjoys the carnal benefits of marriage without the duties of submission required from a wife. Her fortune, indeed, provides the "wages," as Tom later realizes, for his "service" and has for the others before him (720). Nightingale offers a neat solution for Tom to extricate himself from his obligations: "Propose marriage and she will declare off in a moment" (720). In a highly affected letter expressing concern for Lady Bellaston's reputation, Tom asks for her hand: "As your honour is as dear to me as my own, so my sole ambition is to have the glory of laying my liberty at your feet; and believe me when I assure you I can never be made completely happy without you generously bestow on me a legal right of calling you mine forever" (721). Tom's explicit use of "legal" implies his wish to convert Lady Bellaston's status from *feme sole* to *feme covert*, transferring the entirety of her wealth into his hands upon their marriage. The loss of her property, above anything else, is anathema to her independent sensibility. And the style of his writing—which in truth was dictated by the shrewd Nightingale—operates on the opposite emotional level as hers in its transparent artifice. While her letters' style conveys authenticity and immediacy of her emotions, his letter is a studied display of pretended feeling, a feigned honor to restore her reputation as a virtuous wife.

Unsurprisingly, Lady Bellaston detects the hollow presumptuousness of the letter's style and explicitly communicates her revulsion to marriage: "When I read over your serious epistle, I could, from its coldness and formality have sworn that you already had the legal right you mention; nay, that we had for many years composed that monstrous animal a husband and wife" (721). She impugns the sentimentality of marriage, saying that "coldness and formality" define the emotional connection between husband and wife. Amorous passion cannot exist in the strictly constrained institution of marriage, especially in its demands for the wife's domestic seclusion and total financial dependence on the husband. In the libertine framework of sexual freedom, Tom's "proofs of love" (721) in the proposal work as a contradiction. Marriage is a prison where passion dies. Furthermore, she clarifies the limits of her emotional indulgence: "Do you really then imagine me a fool? Or do you fancy yourself capable of so entirely persuading me out of my senses, that I should deliver my whole fortune into your power, in order to enable you to support your pleasures at my expense?" (721). While she may place herself into voluntary abjection for sexual union, marriage would require categorical submission to her husband. Wealth affords choice. She refuses him but adds the familiar postscript: "P.S. I am prevented from revising—Perhaps I have said more than I meant—Come to me at eight this evening" (721). She dismisses his proposal but still seeks to gratify her desire for her lover. By refusing to validate the sentimental mythologizing behind marriage proposals, Lady Bellaston maintains the upper hand in the power dynamic between herself and Tom.

However, Tom doubles down in his response. He is "shocked at [her] suspicion" and asks how she can "treat the most solemn tie of love with contempt" (721). To strengthen the commitment of his marriage proposal, he offers to return "those pecuniary obligations" (721), directly and distastefully indicating the transactional nature of their relationship. It is this final point that turns Lady Bellaston's desire for Tom into hatred: "I see you are a villain; and I despise you from my soul" (722). True to her earlier threat, she can "detest as violently as [she has] loved" (651). Although Tom and Lady Bellaston are very much aware of the implicit financial arrangement between them, Tom's direct and offensive acknowledgment of such an arrangement makes him a "villain." Tom's disingenuous offer is received as a threat: In a 1735 pamphlet titled *The Hardship of the English Laws in Relation to Wives*, Sarah Chapone maintained that marriage puts women in "a worse condition than slavery itself" since, unlike wives, slaves held some rights of redress.[77] This sentiment, while grossly overstated and insensitive in its comparison with enslavement, echoes Lady Bellaston's aversion to marriage as a threat to her independence. In an ironic turn, Lady Bellaston's refusal of Tom's "treatment" for her hysteria cures her "strange infatuation." In parody of hysteria discourse, which promotes marriage as a cure for nervous disorders of women, Tom's proposal effectively moves Lady Bellaston to moderate her desire, but through the opposite means that the medical model has explained. The writings of Anne Finch and Lady Wortley Montagu contest the idea that domesticity liberates women from hysterical symptoms; in fact, marriage may have exacerbated them.[78] Fielding incorporates the rhetoric of the nerve in parody of the expressive structures of medical discourse, structures that legitimize the oppressive institution of marriage, with the life of sexual and economic bondage that define women's realities, a life Lady Bellaston violently rejects.

As I have shown in my reading of Lady Booby's character, passions counterbalanced themselves, rather than being controlled through reason. Action springs from the passions, and Lady Bellaston's progress of feeling drives her motivations and the narrative's plot. The desire for sexual union, once obstructed by her lover, transforms into a desire for vengeance. In *Progress through the Passions*, Haywood theorizes the development of these dangerous passions, a slippery slope beginning with anger:

> Nothing is so violent as anger in its first emotions, it takes the faculties by surprize, and rushes upon the soul like an impetuous torrent, bearing

> down all before it. . . . Should its force continue, it would lose its name, and be no longer anger, but revenge; which, though the worst and most fiend-like propensity of a vicious inclination, is sometimes excited by circumstances, that seem in great measure to alleviate the blackness of it:—repeated and unprovoked insults, friendship and love abused, injuries in our person, our fortune, or reputation, will sour the softest temper, and are apt to make us imagine it is an injustice to our selves, not to retaliate in kind, the ill treatment we receive.[79]

And revenge, "once entertained, is scarce ever extinguished:—it may indeed lie dormant, for a time, but then it easily revives on the least occasion, and blazes out with greater violence than ever. . . . Revenge alone is implacable and eternal, not to be banished by any other passion whatsoever;—the effects of it are the same, invariable in every constitution; and whether the man be phlegmatic or sanguine, there will be no difference in his way of thinking in this point."[80] With Tom's proposal, he manages to injure her "person," "fortune," and "reputation" in one blow. Lady Bellaston's schemes to remove her rival began before Tom's proposal, attempting to arrange a match, then rape, between Sophia and her friend Lord Fellamar. She tests Fellamar's masculine pride, asking with icy contempt, "Are you frightened by the word rape?" (696). By titling this chapter "By which it will appear how dangerous an advocate a lady is when she applies her eloquence to an ill purpose" (696), Fielding directly addresses the immediate danger and power of an impassioned woman. Lady Bellaston shames Fellamar into acquiescence by attacking his masculinity: "Do you think any woman in England would not laugh at you in her heart?" (697). She admits, "you force me to use a strange kind of language," in her support of rape, "to betray [her] sex most abominably" (697), but she believes the desired result of a good marriage match outweighs the darkness of her scheme. Abominably, she normalizes rape as due course in any marriage, stating, "I fancy few of my married acquaintance were ravished by their husbands" (696). Fellamar's attempt to rape Sophia, however, is thwarted when Squire Western bursts into the room. As Simon Dickie has noted, sexual violence in comic works functioned as a plot device; the narrative retains its "happy ending" if the consequences result in the heroine's escape.[81] Sophia's escape from Fellamar saves her from further sexual violence and from falling into the trap of marrying a fiend, orchestrated by Lady Bellaston, clearing the way for Sophia's union with Tom. Truly, in Haywood's words, revenge as "the worst and most fiend-like propensity of a vicious inclination" manifests as unthinkable violence on a woman whom Lady Bellaston once considered under her protection. And returning to Ahern's observation of the paradox of the ideal of romantic love—that the violence experienced through the passions is concomitant with an abject violence on the self—Lady Bellaston redirects this violence onto others in vengeance.

Undeterred, Lady Bellaston directs her "implacable and eternal" vengeance toward Tom, devising a scheme with Fellamar to remove Tom entirely from the country under the pretense of female solidarity and compassion:

> I am thinking, my lord . . . whether it would not be possible for your lordship to contrive some method of having him pressed and sent on board a ship. Neither law nor conscience forbid this project: for the fellow, I promise you, however well drest, is but a vagabond, and as proper as any fellow in the streets to be pressed into the service; and as for the conscientious part, surely the preservation of a young lady from such ruin is a most meritorious act; nay, with regard to the fellow himself, unless he could succeed (which Heaven forbid) with my cousin, it may probably be the means of preserving him from the gallows, and perhaps may make his fortune in an honest way. (761)

Like Lady Booby, she exploits her status as a woman of wealth and high social connections to punish those who injured her pride. Affecting generosity and benevolence for the safety and security of vulnerable young people, Lady Bellaston uses her gender and class position to further her own campaign of revenge.

Lady Bellaston takes her vengeful campaign further with her use of Tom's "love letter." She hands the letter to Di Western as evidence of Tom's infidelity, a document Di calls "a masterpiece of assurance" (763). Writing on the epistolary form in Haywood's novels, Sharon Harrow notes that "as a metonym for the desiring body, the love letter is vulnerable to misinterpretation, exploitation, and scandal."[82] The letter can also serve as a tool for manipulation and exploitation, by the writer, the addressee, or a third party who intercepts it.[83] Lady Bellaston successfully harnesses this power to briefly drive a wedge between Sophia and Tom. Lady Bellaston's ability to manipulate how she and others are seen recalls *The Injur'd Husband*'s Baroness de Tortillée. Jerry Beasley observes that "this woman is a maker of fictions who perverts the storyteller's art by using it to lie, and because she is so skillful her version of the truth threatens to supplant all other possible versions."[84] The Baroness orchestrates a misunderstanding between the two lovers, Montamour and Beauclair, in the same fashion as Lady Bellaston does with Sophia and Tom. The letter stands as an authentic artifact that confirms Tom's infidelity (though he has been, in fact, unfaithful to Sophia throughout the novel, not only with Lady Bellaston but also with Mrs. Waters) and rends the two apart temporarily. But in true Fielding fashion, the true genteel lineage of Tom is revealed as Mr. Allworthy's nephew (rendering him an appropriate candidate for Sophia's hand), Tom begs for Sophia's forgiveness, and the world of the comic novel is set right.

The Baroness is ultimately imprisoned for her crimes and then dies by her own hand, ending "her shameful life."[85] Lady Bellaston suffers no such tragic fate and remains unpunished at the novel's end. With the same public restraint, she made "a formal visit at her return to town, where she behaved to Jones as a perfect stranger, and, with great civility, wished him joy on his marriage" (869). As in *Joseph Andrews*, the power balance is restored through the reaffirmation of the quiet, country gentility in the unification of the Western and Allworthy families. Once again, the failed machinations of the libertine woman drive the comic plot to its happy resolution of domestic harmony.

## DESPISING THE PLEASURES OF LOVE

In *Fielding and the Woman Question*, Angela J. Smallwood argues that the "manly" Fielding was aware of women's issues and featured their social difficulties through his heroines.[86] I argue that the same could be said for the female antagonists in his novels. In *Tom Jones*, Fielding becomes more explicit in what he saw as the deleterious effects of elite women's upbringing. In the opening chapter for book 14 in *Tom Jones*, the narrator demystifies the supposed splendor of the "higher order of mortals," stating that "the highest life is much the dullest, and affords little humour or entertainment," and its characters occupy themselves with ambition or pleasure, wholly "vanity and servile imitation" (649). In this elite circle of people with frivolous pursuits, he exempts women for whom "passion exercises its tyranny," "distinguished by their noble intrepidity" and "a certain superior contempt of reputation" (649). With Lady Bellaston, Fielding attributes her character's vicious behavior to her early education: "Our present women have been taught by their mothers to fix their thoughts only on ambition and vanity, and to despise the pleasures of love as unworthy of their regard; and being afterwards, by the care of such mothers, married without having husbands, they seem pretty well confirmed in the justness of those sentiments" (650). Taught to "despise the pleasures of love" and to "fix their thoughts only on ambition and vanity," daughters displace the natural desire of meaningful love with that of material wealth and ostentation. In their formative years, young ladies learn to repress the natural inclination to choose a partner on the basis of love and affection, redirecting their desire away from its natural course. Therefore, when "passion exercises its tyranny" on these grown ladies and propels them to pursue their love objects in ways beyond what decorum permits, Fielding may respect their "intrepidity" or fearlessness in their honesty to themselves.

Fielding's new brand of realism unsettled his audiences. *The Grub Street Journal* criticized Fielding for presenting low characters with more complexity, such as the sex workers in his satirical play *The Covent Garden Tragedy* (1730).[87] Subverting neoclassical conventions of punishing the bawd and the trull for their wicked ways, he creates figures that elicit a more ambivalent reaction from the audience by framing these characters as fashioned by a society fraught with anxiety regarding women's sexuality. Fielding retains his comedy's moral purpose in his composition of realistic characters in the novels, often framing low comic characters—such as wanton women—as subjects constructed by the dominant discourses of his time. Though Ladies Booby and Bellaston belong to the elite, their sexual appetite categorizes them as belonging to that group of women who violate society's moral values that define women as paragons of virtue. On the one hand, Fielding levels his satire at the impunity that the privileged enjoyed. On the other hand, the novels' appropriation of medical discourse in these women's utterances makes more visible the material realities of that privilege, which take on a completely different color from their male counterparts.

In Fielding's novels and in his own life, he offers the loving companionate marriage, with children as evidence of a healthy sex life, as the palliative measure for unhappiness. Baines identifies "internal reform, love, marriage, and consummation" as resolutions to the social problems in Fielding's novels.[88] However, this is impossible for Ladies Booby and Bellaston, for marriage would mean death to their freedom. While Lady Booby briefly entertains the idea of marrying her footman, Lady Bellaston is clear-eyed on the prison that is marriage. As female libertines, they endeavor to assume the same sexual agency as their male counterparts; this incongruence in its disruption to the established gender hierarchy is deployed for comic effect and culminates in their failures to hinder the happiness of more deserving characters. And yet, with their emotional struggles articulated through their speech and writing shaped by amatory language, Ladies Booby and Bellaston become comic *and* sympathetic subjects. Medical discourse contradicts the Enlightenment ethos of self-determination. Or, more specifically, this self-determination is reserved only for men, as women's physiological experiences always operated within cultural norms and expectations. The hysterical utterances of both women express a verisimilitude of a turbulent emotional life, reaching for liberation denied them.

The science of the nerve is the aperture through which we can observe medicine deploying the familiar narrative of problematic female sexuality, historically grounded in the fear of the female body. Women, defined by their undisciplined passions, dramatize the emotional work of being subject simultaneously to one's physiology and to patriarchal institutions. Fielding, in asking his readers to recognize their overdetermined suffering, points, perhaps, to a more complex understanding of women's happiness.

In chapter 3, I continue my discussion of medicine's essentialist construction of women as frail beings in need of masculine policing and protection within the culture of pregnancy. The women in *Tristram Shandy* and *Peregrine Pickle* insist on bodily autonomy and authority in midwifery; this insistence becomes a source of conflict within the home and within the increasingly clinical, male-dominated area of obstetrics, demonstrating how the maternal body operates as a disruptive resistance to absolute patriarchal control.

# 3

# THE MATERNAL BODY AND OBSTETRIC AUTHORITY IN LAURENCE STERNE'S *TRISTRAM SHANDY* (1759) AND TOBIAS SMOLLETT'S *PEREGRINE PICKLE* (1751)

THE FEMALE BODY'S DISTINCTIVE REPRODUCTIVE features render it a site of disorder, a liminal space between the created and the uncreated. Marilyn Francus traces the associations of the pregnant woman with monstrosity, beginning with Scylla in Homer's *Odyssey*: "encoded as an emblem of lust, the fecund female and her yelping parasitic progeny evoke the seemingly uncontrollable nature of femininity, and not surprisingly, the image functions as a locus of male disgust with, and fear of, sexuality and reproduction."[1] Augustan writing, as a continuation of the early negative readings of fertility, features the womb as embodying emptiness. Susan Gubar has noted the pattern of monstrous maternity from Edmund Spenser's *Faerie Queene* (1590) to Alexander Pope's *Dunciad* (1728–1743) and the accompanying Augustan disgust with female corporeality.[2] In "This Sex Which Is Not One," Luce Irigaray discusses this inscription of the female's "lack" and the "horror of nothing to see."[3] However, Bakhtin sees the womb as an essential constituent of the grotesque body, in which "the very material bodily lower stratum of the grotesque image (food, wine, the genital force, the organs of the body) bears a deeply positive character" in reflecting the universal, the people, materializing the abstract and the ideal into flesh.[4] The English physician William Harvey admires the liminal quality of the womb's egg, calling it "a period of eternity," positioned between the beginning, middle, and end.[5] This tenor of ambivalence of the womb's cultural representations, as both monstrous and cosmic, to be feared and adored, of everything and nothing, is conspicuous in the medical debates regarding human generation, maternal impressions, and parental attribution in the eighteenth century. This ambivalence is also reflected in the culture of pregnancy in which the expecting mother temporarily gains bodily and domestic agency, defended and protected by the women-led expertise of midwifery.

Building on Francus's analysis of the patriarchal fear and disgust associated with female creation and power during pregnancy, this chapter argues that the maternal body looms as a disruptive force and a threat to be vanquished by the increasingly clinical, male-dominated field of midwifery. In Laurence Sterne's *Tristram Shandy* (1759), this struggle begins at conception when Tristram's father, Walter, desires complete control over the conditions surrounding his wife's pregnancy and delivery. Walter's obsession mirrors a broader masculine anxiety present in the literary and medical representations of women's bodies. These depictions are rooted in discursive systems that establish women's physical and emotional frailty based on notions of excess and fluidity, systems constructed to possess women's bodies through knowledge.

Within the field of obstetrics, there exists the masculine desire to gain access to the inaccessible: the womb. In turn, these practitioners produced a body of knowledge that ultimately shows the mutually reinforcing epistemological links between science and patriarchy, in similar ways as menstruation and hysteria theory. As obstetrical science advanced, gender domination in medicine continued to preserve the father's central role in generation, even at the cost of assuming a weak and anxious masculinity. At the center of these debates on parental attribution is the paradoxical negation and affirmation of the mother's role in the production of a grotesque child. Imagined to be essentially frail, vulnerable to external impressions, and at the mercy of her passions, the pregnant woman's body becomes a precious entity to be governed and policed. In the opening chapters of Tobias Smollett's *Peregrine Pickle* (1751), the culture of pregnancy serves as the basis and the target of the novel's satire. Unlike Sterne, Smollett's professional training in medicine and editorial experience with medical writing equipped him with extensive knowledge on the subject. *Peregrine Pickle* also takes up the question of parental attribution in *Tristram Shandy* and engages with several related debates—midwifery, sham practitioners, reading practices—to ultimately discredit women's ways of knowing as manipulative to others and harmful to themselves.

Unlike the linguistic and sexual excesses of Shamela, Lady Booby, and Lady Bellaston, which serve as sources of comic effect and comic irony, the women's pretentions in Sterne's and Smollett's novels do not rise to the point of serious threat for other, more deserving characters; each woman's aspiration for agency is deflated, exposed, or punished at the novel's end, aligning with the comic novel's conservative plot structure in restoring social order and domestic harmony. Rather, the satirical aims of *Tristram Shandy* and *Peregrine Pickle* dispute the long-standing tradition of women's obstetric authority, particularly as the emerging clinical and diagnostic branch of professionalized obstetrics gains more legitimacy, purportedly presenting a path to scientific progress. And yet, as I will demonstrate, the same old rationale of women's essential frailty in theories of menstruation and hysteria is also used to undermine one of the last bastions of female knowledge to further expand and solidify male authority in another arena of cultural life. Both novels, I argue, are informed by masculine anxieties over pregnancy, birthing, and midwifery, as the obstetric authority of women is questioned, ridiculed, and dismissed, resulting in the erasure of the pregnant woman's experience and agency with the ascendancy of clinical medicine.

## LAURENCE STERNE'S *TRISTRAM SHANDY*

Walter Shandy's personification of health presupposes that the soul can truly flourish only within a healthy body: "O blessed health! . . . thou art above all gold and treasure; 'tis thou who enlarges the soul, and openest all its powers to receive instruction and to relish virtue.—He that has thee, has little more to wish for;—and he that is so wretched as to want thee,—wants everything with thee."[6] Unsurprisingly, Tristram's application of Walter's Traducianist principles, the "disaster in the book of embryotic evils" (236), prophesies a life plagued by illness and, by extension, a soul unable to thrive: "I tremble to think what a foundation had been laid for a thousand weaknesses both of body and mind, which no skill of the physician or the philosopher could ever afterwards have set thoroughly to rights" (6). Both father and son are determined that a person's fate hinges on that first act of conception.

Though Walter blames himself for the unfortunate events around his son's birth, Tristram holds both parents accountable: "they were in duty both equally bound to it" (5). Tristram's claim aligns closely with the prevailing theories regarding generation at the time. While the role of the father was mostly focused on conception, it was believed that the mother's emotional and physical state primarily impacted fetal development, delivery, and the child's physical and mental wellbeing. A double urgency appears: A woman's body, by medical definition, was perpetually in a state of unhealthiness, and pregnancy only exacerbated her debilitative condition. William Sermon in *The Ladies Companion; or, The English Midwife* (1671) calls pregnancy "the greatest disease that can afflict women."[7] Writing around the same time as *Tristram Shandy*'s publication, the physician and man-midwife Brudenell Exton characterized pregnancy as a state of illness: "As various symptoms are the consequence of conception, for a woman, during the time of pregnancy, is to be considered as a sick person."[8] For the most favorable outcome, responsibility rested on the father to implant the vitalizing spirit at conception and to ensure the fetus's healthy development through the policing and containment of the mother's body. The womb, in many ways, was a site of contention: How much power do we give to which parent? Which parent is ultimately responsible for a child's apparent inadequacies? Whom to credit? Whom to blame?

### *The Limits of Masculine Control of Knowledge*

As a narrative primarily concerned with the circumstances surrounding a single birth, *Tristram Shandy* is a novel about the masculine desire to access the inaccessible: the operations inside the mother's womb. Tristram inherits Walter's masculine anxieties of ceding control of women's authority in body and knowledge. By writing his autobiography, Tristram embarks on a digressive voyage of self-discovery, with conception as the primary point of departure. And yet, while Mrs. Shandy's body is central to the narrative, readers receive little insight into her own direct experience. This is representative of historical fact, as E. Ann Kaplan has argued that the subjective experience of pregnancy, seldom recorded, can be complicated and contradictory.[9] The novel's absence of women, Ruth Perry asserts, is where the novel's misogyny rests: "Despite the valiant attempts of Ruth Faurot and Leigh Ehlers to demonstrate Mrs. Shandy as a vivid presence and beneficent antidote to the obsessive Shandy men, she and the other women barely exist in the narrative except in their concern for their phallus. As Tristram himself averts, "all the SHANDY FAMILY were of an original character throughout;—I mean the males,—the females had no character at all." Perry contends that the male "marriage between Toby and Trim is the emotional center of the book," also observing that it would be problematic to interpret the Shandy males' vexations as "symptomatic of the cosmic irony of human life," since "the overtones are comic rather than tragic, and women are the butts of the joke."[10]

While I agree with Perry that women are largely absent in *Tristram Shandy*, this absence, I believe, indicates the degree of power women wield in the narrative, the kind of epistemological power men fear and find frustrating. The near absence of women's direct experience in a novel about a man's birth and about men's emotions implies a reluctant acknowledgment of women's agency and authority in matters regarding their bodies. Walter's frustrations with his wife and their servant Susannah stem from the women's refusal to recognize his authority in what they perceive as an exclusively female domain of knowledge. And in writing a story about a birth that prominently features male characters while leaving female figures on the periphery, Tristram can only write within the epistemological limitations of masculine understanding, no matter how far the story line may wander.

At the time of Tristram's birth, Mrs. Shandy's absence from the narrative is conspicuous. Although we receive no insight on her direct experience, the collective power of the women in the household is raised through the event of birth. Her body may not be visible, but it remains a perennial presence in the backdrop of household conversation and as the source of the writer's existence. While a single woman's bodily experience is omitted from the narrative, the women's collective presence situates them all at the center of the story. Mrs. Shandy's labor takes place offstage, while Walter and Toby discourse on "TIME and ETERNITY" (151), an apt topic during a birth, given the womb's associations with what Harvey called "a period of eternity." Francus interprets Mrs. Shandy's bodily absence as containment as a result of the masculine inscription of the ideal femininity, a body stripped of both sex and social authority, thereby excluding women from her own generative powers.[11] However, the communal quality of labor and birth, I offer as a counterpoint, absorbs and embodies Mrs. Shandy's absence and increases female authority in the household, even for a short while. The only person who speaks for Mrs. Shandy is her maid Susannah, who curtly responds to Walter's inquiry of her mistress's condition that she is "as well as can be expected" (230). Walter begrudges women's solidarity during pregnancy and childbirth, a "puzzling riddle": "from the very moment the mistress of the house is brought to bed, every female in it, from my lady's gentlewoman down to the cinder-wench, becomes an inch taller for it; and give themselves more airs upon that single inch, than all their inches put together" (227). The temporary state of pregnancy and the period of childbirth elevates the status of women in the family household, a status men have previously accepted.[12] The English midwife Elizabeth Nihell, in a powerful rebuke against male midwifery, asserted that the art of obstetrics is exclusive to women and that the fashion for male practice is a perversion of the "natural order of things."[13] What is more, female midwives rely on their woman-specific embodiment and sympathy to care for birthing mothers: "midwives, beside their personal experience, being sometimes themselves the mothers of children, have a kind of intuitive guide within themselves, the original organ of conception, itself pregnant, in more cases than that, with a strong instinctive influence on the mind and actions of the sex."[14] Nevertheless, Walter resents this masculine inaccessibility. Susannah's brusque remark "as well as can be expected" either could presume Walter's understanding of the birth event or could be a cutting remark on his ignorance. Of course, he has no idea, and this epistemological lack decenters him, relegating him to the periphery of reproductive control.

### *The Political Stakes of Parental Attribution*

In the century preceding the publication of *Tristram Shandy*, debates concerning procreation often centered on the mother's role in mediating the link between children and the patriarchal source, be it God, king, or father. John Locke, who had some medical experience, suggests in *Two Treatises of Government* (1690) that "God says, *Honour thy Father and Mother*; but our Author . . . leaves out *thy Mother* quite, as little serviceable to his purpose."[15] Interested in the forces shaping political rhetoric, Locke argues against absolute monarchical power if the role of the mother is dismissed—admitting that her active capacity in generation would suggest that the father (or king) would not have a fundamental right to sole control. Locke's case for generation draws from and reshapes Aristotelian and Galenic theories, insisting that pregnancy, not the sperm's fertilization of the egg, shapes the female matter into a child. Locke's emphasis is on the process of fetal development, arguing that the embryo's growth in the mother determines the child's outcome.[16] Thomas Hobbes makes a similar argument in both *De Cive* (1642) and *Leviathan* (1651), claiming that paternity alone cannot be the definitive justification for the basis of sovereignty because "the originall Dominion over *children* belongs to the *Mother*. . . . The birth followes the belly."[17] In contrast, Sir Robert Filmer's *Patriarcha* (1680), the most recognized work on patriarchal political theory of the time, was fundamentally organized around the exclusion of the mother. Defending the sovereignty of kings, Filmer claimed that "the law which enjoins obedience to kings is delivered in the terms of 'honour thy father' . . . as if all power were originally in the father."[18] He addresses the father's sole capacity in generation: "We know that God at the creation gave sovereignty to the man over the woman, as being the nobler and principal agent in generation."[19] Filmer's use of "generation" emphasized the link between the child and the father, the first source of patriarchal value. Ludmilla Jordanova observes that the shift from the earlier term "generation" to "reproduction" to describe the production of human offspring signals the collapsing of difference from the patriarchal system to a maternal one.[20] The contrast between these accounts of generation and male dominion parallels the scientific debates of parental attribution and maternal impressions. The central threat these debates challenged or affirmed is the physiology of paternity and, by extension, reigning theories of patriarchal dominance in social and political life. Parental attribution to the father informed social structures. For example, until the passage of the Infant Custody Act in 1839, which gave mothers the right to keep or visit their children after divorce or separation, English common law granted the father sole custody of children and even the guardianship order after his death.[21] As extensions of the father, children were considered possessions to be disposed of as he saw fit, even posthumously.

### *Masculine Anxiety as Instrument of Gender Domination in Medicine*

Considering how paternity affirms dominant masculine selfhood, Walter's desperation to claim total control over his role in Tristram's conception seems warranted. During the visitation dinner, Walter could hardly contain his excitement when Doctor Kysarcius makes the provocative claim that "the mother is not of kin to her child" (262), as determined by the case of the Duke of Suffolk. Juliet McMaster describes Walter's deep investment in sole paternal attribution in conception as a "severe case of ovary-envy"; he seems to draw no pleasure in intercourse ("Not a jot"), but he desires to physically carry out and receive recognition for the operations of conception, pregnancy, and birth. McMaster continues, "He wants the child to be all his; and since he can't quite achieve this, his next choice (like the podalic inversion if he can't have a caesarean) is to reduce the mother's role to as near nothing as possible."[22] Walter's masculine anxiety drives his effort to erase the mother. Mark Breitenberg points out that while "anxiety is both a negative effect that leads us to patriarchy's own internal discord, . . . it is also an instrument (once properly contained, appropriated or returned) of its perpetuation."[23]

William Harvey's *Exercitationes de generatione animalium* (1651) threatened to contravene theories that supported knowledge of male dominion, serving as a case of how masculine anxiety acts as an instrument in preserving masculine dominance in medical discourse. Finding no semen in the uterus after intercourse, Harvey determines that fertilization occurred without the semen's contact with the egg, departing from Aristotle's and Galen's views on conception. Aristotle believed that the semen activated the menstrual clot with a soul, with the woman supplying only the matter in which the semen shaped the child. For Aristotle, the woman's capacity as material cause gave her the right as a parent. However, the man's contribution that gives the motion and direction of the offspring's formation endowed him with the right as the primary progenitor.[24] Aristotle explains, "The female body always provides the material, the male that which fashions it. . . . While the body is from the female, it is the soul that is from the male."[25] Galen, while disputing Aristotle's theory in assigning procreative seed to the woman, concurred with Aristotle's assertion of the woman's subordinate role. In Galenic anatomy, women were seen as imperfect versions of men due to their colder bodies, resulting in internal reproductive organs for warmth. As a result, the seed produced by women's reproductive organs was deficient in quality compared to the seed produced by the perfect organs of men.[26] Galen's corrections to Aristotelian theory, on the surface, may appear to exhibit medical advancement by acquired knowledge. Yet, scientific progress only continued to uphold existing gendered hierarchies. Even when faced with the possibility of equal, or perhaps sole, parental attribution to the mother, male physicians like William Harvey proposed speculations that preserved the father's central role in generation.

Harvey's discovery of the semen's distance from the egg compelled him to admit his loss at determining how fertilization occurs. Still, he conjured scenarios that realigned the female with matter and the male with the power of spirit. He suggested that the semen might work like a magnet: "the woman after contact with the spermatic fluid in coitus, seems to receive influence and to become fecundated without the cooperation of any sensible corporeal agent, in the same way as iron touched by a magnet is endowed with its powers and can attract other iron to it."[27] The second scenario suggested that the semen acted like a disease, spreading through contagion: "epidemic, contagious, and pestilential diseases scatter their seeds, and are propagated at a distance through the air, or by some 'fomes' producing diseases like themselves, in bodies of a different nature, and in a hidden fashion silently multiply . . . themselves by a kind of generation."[28] His final theory depicted the semen as a God-like creator capable of miracles: "What is this transitory thing which is neither to be found remaining, nor touching, nor contained, as far as the sense inform us, and yet works with the highest intelligence and foresight, beyond all art; and which, even after it has vanished, renders eggs prolific . . . and makes the hen herself fruitful before she has yet produced any germs of eggs, and this too so suddenly, as it were said by the Almighty, 'Let there be progeny,' and straight it is so? . . . In the generation of things is seen most excellent, the eternal and almighty God."[29] In each case, seminal fluid is considered to be the vitalizing power in the womb. Harvey, like Aristotle and Galen before him, gives primary parental attribution to the father.

Harvey's treatment of the egg may appear to break with medical tradition, but his work still reinforced long-standing views of gender systems of masculine domination. Keller concludes, "the implicit project of *de Generatione* to aggrandize the father and reduce the mother coalesces, for Harvey makes the offspring the exclusive image of the father, constructed on the near denial of the mother."[30] Ultimately, Harvey's embryological theories view the mother's role as briefly active, for she generates the egg but is then disconnected from it. This brief agency is integral to the characteristic of male roles in conception, that in providing the egg while being separated from it, the mother enables the father's capacity to be imagined as God-like with the egg acting on his own masculine authority. Operating for a brief interval between the shot of "divine semen" and the independent embryo's development, the mother becomes the subject for the definition of male selfhood. She is the vessel through which the father reproduces himself and the sanctuary of nutrition for the embryo. Keller observes, "The mother in Harvey's theory serves biologically the roles that she was beginning to serve socially in the emerging bourgeois household. When Harvey therefore looks into the 'heart of the mystery' of generation, he sees what surrounds him: 'self-sufficing and independent' males and the females whose function it is to promote them."[31] In this line of reasoning, the womb is the site of domestic politics; the womb is imagined as a home in which the father is the sole contributor—if we think of the sperm as income—and the mother's responsibility is to passively, gratefully receive his contribution in acceptance, affirmation, and promotion of his authority. For men, in the mysterious universe of the womb, the semen and the egg dramatize the father's and mother's biological roles in the domestic hierarchy. Similar to theories of menstruation and hysteria, gender roles are naturalized at the cellular level, reproduced and repeated in the cycle of birth. And yet, the women in *Tristram Shandy* disrupt the myths of biological and domestic essentialism. Women fiercely guard obstetrical epistemologies that belong exclusively to them, and the pregnant mother, by insisting on a female midwife and rejecting a caesarean delivery, refuses to yield power and authority to the father in matters regarding labor and birth.

While Walter's exhortations had little effect on the women in his household, his insistence that his authority on generative matters be acknowledged did not come from a vacuum. Generative powers in the rhetoric of embryology are figuratively conferred to men, granting physiological ground for the source and construction of human identity. Both Harvey and his contemporary surgeon Nathaniel

Highmore incorporated vitalist principles in their embryology theories, constructing a system of representation that bestows agency on the father. Harvey posits that the embryo has an inborn vital spirit that governs its growth and development.[32] Highmore takes this concept further by suggesting that the spiritual element, the "soul playing the skillful workman," is carried to the ovum through the semen. Successful generation only occurs when the soul accompanies the sperm in its travels to the egg. Highmore explains that once the father's soul becomes "intent on propagation and multiplying her self into another Individuum . . . [she] diffuseth her self into the . . . parting sperm" and makes it "prolifical," "which coming into a convenient receptacle, where these Atomes may repose; being moved only by that soul which accompanied them, and from which they received their orders and commands, are soon settled into their proper places, and become a perfect Individuum *of that Species*."[33] Felicity Nussbaum notes this "profound historical contradiction": "Eighteenth-century Englishmen largely defined themselves, sexually and materially as fully outside the scope of the maternal yet eager to intervene with it."[34] Walter embodies this contradiction in his fervor to enter the maternal by occupying intellectual space through abstract speculating and citing ancient and modern male authorities, such as the French philosopher René Descartes, the Italian alchemist and physician Coglionissimo Borri, the Danish anatomist Thomas Bartholin, and the English physician John Burton. McMaster calls Walter a misogynist, "but the source of his misogyny is curious, and intricately developed. He is moved less by dislike of women than by envy. . . . He longs to do the whole job of procreation by himself."[35] In the masculine ideal and for Walter, the model for love is "rational . . . without mother—where Venus had nothing to do" (473–475).

Obviously, Walter's fantasy of asexual reproduction is impossible, so he imagines scenarios that enable him to take primary responsibility for the origins and shape of his son's identity, starting with what he viewed as a failed generation at Tristram's conception: "But alas! My Tristram's misfortunes began nine months before he ever came into the world" (7).[36] According to the English physician Erasmus Darwin, the father's thoughts during sex or orgasm "may so affect this secretion by irratative or sensitive association . . . as to cause the production of similarity of form and of features, with the distinction of sex."[37] In those critical moments, the father must concentrate on an image in his mind to ensure the mental and physical health of his progeny. It is no wonder, then, that Walter and Tristram attribute Mrs. Shandy's "unseasonable question" during coitus as a catastrophic event: "Pray, my dear . . . have you not forgot to wind up the clock?" (5). A "slave" to "extreme exactness," Walter winds up the clock on the first Sunday night of every month before lying with his wife. In Lockean terms, due to "an unhappy association of ideas," Mrs. Shandy soon associated the sound of the winding of the clock with sex. Walter's rare act of spontaneity occasioned this question, interrupting him and thereby resulting in his animal spirits being, in Walter's words, "dispers'd, confused, confounded, scattered, and sent to the devil" (236). And, as a consequence of the animal spirits' poor distribution, as reported by Tristram through his Uncle Toby, who overheard Walter complain "oft" and "heavily" (7), the homunculus, the fully formed microscopic human being in the womb, suffered without the safe guidance of the animal spirits: "my little gentleman had got to his journey's end miserably spent;—his muscular strength and virility worn down to a thread;—his own animal spirits ruffled beyond description,—and that in this sad disorder'd state of nerves, he had laid down a prey to sudden starts, or a series of melancholy dreams and fancies for nine long, long months together" (6). This "shared language of suffering and distress" between men—in this case, between Toby and Walter, and then Toby and Tristram, as Breitenberg explains, is "largely a discourse articulated and played out between men, a way for men to confirm their identity."[38] Tristram inherits his father's anxious masculinity and frames it in such a way that relies on scientific discourse to assert his identity onto the fetus.

Tristram's vivid description of the homunculus's perilous and solitary expedition mimics the figurative language of scientific reasoning and discourse that relies on literary devices such as personification and metaphor.[39] Going against the historical tradition of culture and science denying the fetus a personhood, Tristram creates a whole person at the time of conception, complete with sex assignment, social status, feelings, and the capacity to dream and imagine.[40] The emotional effect of this personification on the reader enlarges the enormity of the mother's supposed crimes. In Walter's thinking (and later adopted by his son), his wife's "unseasonable question" triggered a chain of events that indelibly shaped Tristram to be weak and sickly. Although the fault lies with the mother as the source of imperfect generation, parental attribution, within the confines of the womb, lies entirely on the father as the sole contributor of sperm, the "Fruit of Life," the "vivid stream."[41] This reasoning, in which the mother can be both responsible (through her speech) and vindicated (in her passivity as the vessel) reflects the father's desire for complete reproductive control, eager to claim responsibility for the outcome of the fetus, even at the cost of embodying a frail and fragile masculinity.

Walter's advanced age also supports his primacy in parental attribution. Upon learning that Susannah had mistakenly given the curate the name "Tristram" instead of "Trismegistus," Walter retreats to the fishpond to reflect on his troubles. In the chapter mock-heroically titled "My Father's Lamentation," Walter woefully admits to the damage his older body has inflicted on the fetus: "produced into being, in the decline of thy father's days—when the powers of his imagination and of his body were waxing feeble—when radical heat and radical moisture, the elements which should have temper'd thine, were drying up; and nothing left to found thy stamina in, but negations" (236). Walter believed his aging body (Tristram reveals to his readers that his father was "being somewhere between fifty and sixty years of age"; 8), with its concomitant weakening of mind, is partly to blame for the "embryotic evils" that have fallen on Tristram's head. While the serious application of humoral theory in medicine was waning in the eighteenth century, its beliefs persisted in the popular imagination, evidenced in Walter's language when describing his body's "radical heat" and "radical moisture." As I explain in chapter 1, humoral theory posits that men are naturally hot and dry, while women are cool and wet. Heat, the most positive of these qualities, was the vigor in the body that could most easily transform one type of fluid into another. Heat was also believed to rise instinctively to the brain, explaining why men were more rational than women.[42] Walter's "radical heat" and "radical moisture" were "drying up" with age. Old age implied a lack of vigor, constituting a "horrid frost" that drained "vigorous heat" from the male body.[43] Walter acknowledges that his attempt to "found" his fetus's "stamina," or its healthy growth in the womb stimulated by powerful physical effort, was based on "negations," on denial of his own potency. In other words, he deluded himself into thinking that his constitution was strong enough to conceive a healthy child. In Karen Harvey's study of eighteenth-century erotic culture, she notes the pervasive cultural assumption of older men's impotence. The erotic book *Arbor Vitae; or, The Natural History of the Tree of Life* (1732) describes older men as "subject to become weak and flaccid, and want support."[44] The pornographic *Teague-root Display'd* explains how these old men, in attempting to "keep the Electrical Embers in some tolerable degree of Heat . . . sometimes . . . condescend to discover their Posteriors, and have them heartily flogg'd by their female Servants."[45] Flogging was seen as another means of treating assumed elderly impotence: "some Gardeners have thought of splintring them up with *Birchen Twigs*, which has seemed of some Service for the present, tho' the Plants have very soon come to the same, or more drooping State than before."[46] Pathetic and futile, these measures could not stymie the decay that age wrought. Writers considered sexual arrangements between older men, "greybearded dotards, frozen with age," and younger women, full of "the amorous fire, and vivacity of ardent and passionate youth," as an immoral social embarrassment.[47] Male readers are advised to woo women in their youth, because when "grown feeble with age, our feet will no longer carry us to their temples."[48] These cultural ideas of aging men's inadequacy to "found" a healthy fetus at conception help to confirm Walt's responsibility.

## *Reclaiming Mrs. Shandy*

Roy Porter's label of Mrs. Shandy as a "bovine mother" needs reconsideration.[49] While Walter is certainly vexed with his wife's passive indifference to his proposals for breeching Tristram, his exasperation is not limited to her alone: Susannah,

Obadiah, Dr. Slop, and even Walter's gentler brother Toby have been subjected to his splenetic humor. Mrs. Shandy, in matters unrelated to her, lets her husband take the lead. But when it came to decisions involving her own body, she stands firm. Her insistence on calling an established London man-midwife, and then her own midwife, over Dr. Slop demonstrates her autonomy and independence from her husband.

Mrs. Shandy deserves credit for not being as dull-witted as some readers may believe, even if she knows little of Socratic philosophy. After an hour and a half of arguing with her as a "Christian," then as a "Philosopher," Walter can only attribute his wife's intransigence to her lack of intelligence, that she lacks the mental capacity to see his perspective: "Cursed luck . . . for a man to be master of one of the finest chains of reasoning in nature,—and have a wife at the same time with such a head-piece, that he cannot hang up a single inference within side of it, to save his soul from destruction" (117). In the spirit of Menippean satire, her refusal to engage in verbal and intellectual combat with Walter, the *philosophus gloriosus*, which results in his comic frustration, demonstrates how well she knows her husband (it would be a futile waste of time), and her grounded nature throws Walter's systematizing follies into comic relief. Tristram notes, "It was a consuming vexation to my father, that my mother never asked the meaning of a thing she did not understand.—That she is not a woman of science, my father would say—is her misfortune—but she might ask a question.—My mother never did" (378). If Mrs. Shandy were a "woman of science," she would strive to fill the gaps of her knowledge with questions for her husband. This implies that Walter sees himself as the intellectual authority in their marriage and expects to have all the answers for her. This exchange would affirm Walter's sense of self-worth and superiority, which is heavily grounded in his presumed intelligence. However, because his wife refuses to engage in scholarly activities, he does not receive this reinforcement for his ego. In a way, Mrs. Shandy's indifference is an act of agency; she refuses to give Walter any access to her mental processing, and therefore he cannot influence her thinking in any way. He has no control over any of this, which results in comic frustration.

When Mrs. Shandy becomes pregnant, Walter increasingly scrutinizes and polices his wife's mental and emotional state, concerned with how it could potentially influence the fetus. Jacques Gélis explains in his anthropological study of childbirth that most people in early modern Europe believed a pregnant woman had "a melancholy cast of mind, full of sorrowful ideas," which negatively affects the fetus.[50] This also contradicts the belief that pregnancy can cure the hysterical woman, which I discussed in chapter 2. Inconsistent with both assumptions, Mrs. Shandy is neither melancholic nor hysterical. Her temperament is rather balanced: "A temperate current of blood ran orderly through her veins in all months of the year, and in all critical moments both of the day and night alike; nor did she superinduce the least heat into her humors from the manual effervescencies of devotional tracts, which having little or no meaning in them, nature is oft times obliged to find one" (486). Even when reading religious tracts meant to inspire devotional passion, Mrs. Shandy raises no enthusiasm. So as far as the narrative shows, Mrs. Shandy's blood ran in orderly fashion, with the exception of the labor (which occurs offstage) and her fights with Walter over who would be attending her: "What battles did she fight with me, and what perpetual storms about the midwife. . . . What a teasing life did she lead herself, and consequently her foetus too, with that nonsensical anxiety of hers about lying in town?" (236). For Walter, Mrs. Shandy's self-advocacy in contradiction to her husband's demands needlessly upsets her, and he believes that her self-inflicted emotional distress could potentially harm the child.

Given the discourse on maternal impressions at the time, Walter's frustrations with his wife and his fear for his child's development seem to be justified. Paul-Gabriel Boucé has noted the "epistemological haze" surrounding the maternal impressions debates in the eighteenth century. The most bitter dispute transpired between two doctors from the Royal College of Physicians, Daniel Turner and James Augustus Blondel. A surgeon in England, Turner published *De morbis cutaneis: A Treatise of Diseases Incident to the Skin* in 1714, known as the first English dermatology text but also for the debate on maternal impressions it provoked. In a chapter on birthmarks, Turner explained what he called "that Faculty of the sensitive Soul called Phansy or Imagination" as a biological function that rested in the brain through nervous fluid in response to stimuli. The chapter, titled "Of Spots and Marks of a diverse Resemblance, imprest upon the Skin of the Foetus, by the Force of the Mother's Fancy; with some Things premis'd, of the strange and almost incredible Power of Imagination, more especially in pregnant Women," defended the indelible impact of maternal impressions, that "powerful events during a woman's pregnancy gave rise to malformation of the offspring."[51] He admits, however, that he could not explain this claim, writing, "how these strange Alterations should be wrought, or the Foetus cut, wounded and maimed, as if the same were really done with a Weapon, whilst the Mother is unhurt, and merely by the Force of her Imagination, is, I must confess ingenuously, . . . Supra Captum, i.e. above my Understanding."[52] James Augustus Blondel, a Parisian educated at the University of Leiden and a noted member of the College of Physicians of London, responded virulently to Turner's claims: "What can be more scandalous, and provoking, than to suppose, that those whom God Almighty has endow'd, not only with so many charms, but also with an extraordinary Love and Tenderness for their Children, instead of answering the End they are made for, do bread [*sic*] Monsters by the Wantonness of their Imagination?"[53] Blondel, an anti-imaginationist, casted doubt over the cases cited from medical antiquity and claimed that the infant lived "in a state of neutrality," unaffected by the mother's feelings.[54] Notwithstanding the fury of the debates, Boucé concludes his short history by observing that "whether to the imaginationist or the anti-imaginationists, women appeared as the frail and wayward instrument of procreation, the consenting victim of her wild fancy, a creature in turn reified and deified by Man."[55] Julia Epstein notes the same gender domination discourse in the debates, saying, "What is most striking is that Turner's imaginationist view, which attributed monstrous births to maternal impressions, and Blondel's preformationist view, which argued that the maternal role was merely to house the developing fetus, similarly negated the agency of pregnant women."[56] The debates clarified that women bore the responsibility during pregnancy and that their imagination's potential excesses must be policed. The dominant belief of the woman's natural biological inability for imaginative self-restraint justified her containment and surveillance as a social and moral imperative. While Toby remarks that his sister-in-law "submitted with the greatest patience" and "never utter[ed] a fretful word," Walter insists that "she fumed inwardly . . . and that . . . was ten times worse for the child" (236). Whether Mrs. Shandy's disagreement with her husband manifested as "perpetual storms" or internal fuming, her emotional imbalance and excess were perceived as potentially harming her fetus.

### *The Paradoxical Negation and Confirmation of the Mother's Agency in Generation*

Walter, cognizant that his advanced age and declining vitality worked against the production of a healthy child, directs his energies toward governing his wife's body. Given the prevailing popular and medical discourse that attributed a baby's intellectual or physical disability to the mother, Walter's desperation appears grounded. It is important to note that disability at this time was synonymous with deformity, and I am referring to its usage here as a historical construct.[57] The causes of defects were central to eighteenth-century debates about each parent's role in generation, especially in the wars between the preformationists and epigenicists, and Marie-Hélène Huet has written on the ways teratology, or the scientific study of congenital abnormalities and formations, arose from these debates.[58] The seventeenth-century French physician Claude Quillet writes of the mother's imaginative powers in his poem *The Callipaed; or, The Art of Creating Fair Children* (1749): "The spirits descending from the brain mingle in the womb with the prolific [child-making] essence and penetrate it through and through; there they imprint with invincible force the same images by which they have themselves been struck." Quillet illustrates his point with the metaphor of baking bread: "Thus in a baker's trough, the flour mixed with warm water and set in motion by the yeast, swells up into one single mass; if the baker sets a hand to it, he can make all different kinds of cake of many different shapes: so in women, ideas make the same sort of impressions on the foetus."[59] Even Voltaire reluctantly admits, "This passive imagination in easily disturbed minds can sometimes pass on to children the clear signs of an impression received by the mother. There are innumerable examples of this, and the author of this article has seen some so striking that he would be denying the evidence of his own eyes if he were to doubt it."[60] John Maubray, not a trained doctor but the author of the popular *The Female Physician* (1724), places significant responsibility for these misadventures on the pregnant woman herself: "She ought discreetly to suppress all *Anger*, *Passion*, and other *Perturbations* of Mind, and avoid entertaining too *serious* or *melancholick Thoughts*; since all *such* tend to impress a *Depravity* of Nature upon the Infant's *Mind*, and *Deformity* on its *Body*."[61] Fielding has drawn from the maternal impression debates as a plot device: Joseph Andrews's strawberry-shaped birthmark on his chest is the stamp of his mother's own cravings for strawberries during pregnancy, marking the genetic link between mother and son through the mother's imagination and desires. While birthmarks were a benign symptom of the mother's condition, the production of deformed children was most attributed to the perverse female mind, seen as a sign of contaminated maternity. In short, a healthy birth was attributed to the father's vitality, while deformity was blamed on the mother's pathological physical and mental weakness.

In the latter half of the seventeenth century, there was a growing urgency, particularly among people in higher stations, regarding the need to prevent the dangers of labor and to preserve the mother's life, as dramatized here by Walter's overbearing concern. The regimen for regulating and monitoring pregnant women was based on the belief of their essential frailty, with practices such as immobilization and bleeding at the slightest provocation being standard methods to ensure the safety of both the expectant mother and fetus. Gélis writes, "The result was doubtless a passage from insufficient precautions to an ill-considered protectiveness, with no benefit to the woman, left at the mercy of the slightest false step or the most trivial cold. Dulled reflexes, faintings at the slightest provocation, reduced resistance to pain: this heralds the 'age of the vapours,' convulsions, and panic in childbirth."[62] Walter, in his attempt to control every possible contingency, relies on the knowledge he has gleaned from his books. His logic, of course, is faulty; believing that the soul resides in the brain, near the medulla oblongata, Walter concludes that the "violent compression and crush" of the head through the birth canal by "nonsensical method of bringing [children] into the world by that part foremost" risks damaging the delicate soul (119). His concern may also stem from his first son's outcome, as there is some speculation that Tristram's older brother, Bobby, may have an intellectual disability.[63] After contemplating the dangers of natural delivery, Walter callously determines that "it accounted for the eldest son being the greatest blockhead in the family" (120). Bobby's condition may be the reason why Walter presses his wife for a caesarean delivery, which (in his mind) would reduce the pressure on the infant's skull during a vaginal delivery. While physicians and man-midwives held differing perspectives on delivery, there was nearly unanimous agreement on avoiding caesarean surgery until after the mother's death. This is unsurprising, given that the mortality rate for caesarean delivery without proper anesthesia was a staggering 70 percent.[64] The man-midwife Sir Fielding Ould vehemently condemned the practice as a "detestable, barbarous, illegal piece of inhumanity."[65] Once Walter broaches the topic with his wife, she "turn[ed] pale as ashes at the very mention of it" (121). Compared to the major male characters in the novel, Mrs. Shandy barely speaks. Here, her body becomes the medium for expression, a meaning so clearly articulated through the blanching of her face that even Walter drops the subject. Her silence holds more significance than any utterance, which coheres with the novel's major theme of the failure of language. The panoply of blank pages, black pages, missing chapters, asterisks and dashes, and aposiopesis gesture to Sterne's view that communication is expressed more sincerely through gesture and sympathetic identification. For Walter, the look of fear from his wife does more to end the conversation than spoken dialogue.

If Walter had failed in his role during conception, he believed that his wife's behavior during the pregnancy might, as he claims, "have set all things to rights" (236). However, considering the available models of women's health and pregnancy, this appears to be impossible. Using the language of Galenic medicine, Walter portrays his wife as a careless mother, paying little attention to "her evacuations and repletions . . . and the rest of her non-naturals" (239). Treatment of pregnant women in the long eighteenth century included humoralism's nonnatural factors on health, or the basis of health and disease prevention not inherent in the body, including air, food and drink, exercise and rest, sleep, retention and evacuation of wastes, and perturbations of the mind and emotions. Maubray insisted that the mother preserve domestic harmony in her household: "there never ought so much as a *Cloud* to appear in [her] *Conjugal Society*; since all such unhappy *Accidents* strongly affect the growing *Infant*."[66] In 1668, the French obstetrician François Mauriceau characterized pregnancy as "a rough Sea" and advised pregnant women "to be careful to overcome and moderate her Passions, as not to be excessive angry; and above all, that she be not afrighted; nor that any melancholy news be suddenly told her," because she might miscarry.[67] The French man-midwife F. A. Deleurye recommended a calm environment for the pregnant woman, since she is "naturally inclined to anger and bad temper, more so than at other times."[68] Alexander Hamilton, professor of midwifery at Edinburgh University, warned in his 1781 *Treatise of Midwifery* against "crowds, confinement, every situation which renders [pregnant women] under any disagreeable restriction . . . and whatever disturbs either the body or mind."[69] The man-midwife John Grigg explained that miscarriage could arise from "the indulgence of violent passions, a mode of living inconsistent with the order and simplicity of nature, a view of objects in distress or in imminent danger, the hearing of dreadful accounts, or reading melancholy stories, in short, whatever else can injure the body or disturb the mind."[70] Passions could potentially cause miscarriage, so it was crucial that the pregnant woman be kept calm. However, a contradiction arises when this treatment is imposed on the same leaky bodies that were medically defined as always in excess and in loss of control. As I have explained in chapters 1 and 2, self-possession, though a virtue held in high regard for women, was difficult or impossible to master, at least according to medical belief. For a pregnant woman, it is even more challenging to control her emotions. This idea directly contradicts the belief that pregnancy was one of the effective treatments for hysteria, since the womb is no longer running amok in the woman's body. In 1747, John Henry Mauclerc refuted Blondel's treatise in *Dr. Blondel Confuted; or, The Ladies Vindicated*.[71] Mauclerc's subtitle, *The Ladies Vindicated*, uncovers the principal trouble in these debates: the perception of pregnant women as beings capable of rational thought. The discourse on maternal impressions revealed that the center of responsibility for pregnancy rested with women and that female interiority signified excess requiring monitoring and regulation.

Whether the mother gave vent to or internally suppressed her emotion, practitioners believed that her emotional state would adversely disrupt healthy fetal development. The argument here is that if she was not vocalizing her emotional excess, she must be keeping it pent up—which, according to the hydraulic model, can lead to a disastrous obstruction in the mind and body. As a woman, Mrs. Shandy makes it impossible for Tristram to recover from the injuries sustained in the act of conception. The attribution granted to the mother in fetal (and subject) formation for the child is only granted and affirmed in the production of a grotesque child, paradoxically negating and confirming the mother's agency in generation.

## TOBIAS SMOLLETT'S *PEREGRINE PICKLE*

Like *Tristram Shandy*, masculine anxiety in Smollett's *Peregrine Pickle* (1751) drives the representations of pregnant bodies, with Smollett's satire placed firmly on the culture of pregnancy that grants women brief power over spaces, their bodies, and men. Smollett's earlier medical training, short stint as a man-midwife, and editorial work on his friend William Smellie's obstetric volumes inform his satire of the culture that depends on the private knowledge of women.[72] Unlike Sterne's novel, which grapples with the definitive answer to the question of parental attribution in its sustained attention to conception, *Peregrine Pickle* seems to offer a resolution to the impressionist debates between Turner and Blondel. Smollett's novel envisions the destructive (yet comic) ramifications of women's full and unquestioned agency based on the supposed supremacy of their experiential knowledge. With conception not featured at all in Smollett's novel, the ambiguities regarding genetic inheritance in *Tristram Shandy* are fully realized in the negative vision of maternal attribution in *Peregrine Pickle* with the monstrous mother, Sally Pickle.

What follows is the hypothetical synthesis of humoralism and Hobbesian and Lockean perspectives of the mother's active capacity in shaping her children: Sally's sanguine temperament is inherited by her son Peregrine, forming his character, which Jerry Beasley describes to be "compulsively greedy, opportunistic, profligate, promiscuous, predatory."[73] Perry's character is predicted by his mother's behavior during her pregnancy, a period in which she exploits the culture that reveres and respects the mysteries of gravidity. The attribution granted to Sally in Perry's subject formation is granted and affirmed in the production of a temperamentally imperfect child. However, I argue for a more complex reading, that the masculine homosocial relationships in the novel have more influence in the shaping of Perry's character, especially when we consider the generic conventions of the ramble novel.

*Peregrine Pickle* engages with the debates related to the culture of pregnancy and ways of knowing. Smollett, drawing from his own knowledge of medicine and his experience with editing obstetric tracts, dramatizes the vulnerability of Mrs. Grizzle to undegreed practitioners like Nicholas Culpeper. Smollett criticizes the authorial arrogance of men like Culpeper who publish books for the public, as well as the aspirational autodidactic abilities of women like Mrs. Grizzle who consume such books. These vignettes reveal Smollett's elitism but also betray an anxiety toward the idea of women assuming control over their own knowledge of a subject increasingly believed to belong only to men with diagnostic expertise. And to continue this thread of questioning epistemological authority, the episode of the newly married Mrs. Grizzle, now Mrs. Trunnion, and her phantom pregnancy cautions readers of the consequences of stubbornly refusing the superior expertise of male midwives and the overreliance of women's ways of knowing. Ultimately, *Peregrine Pickle*'s representations of pregnancy reify the troubling consequences of women's bodily and epistemological agency.

## *Sally Pickle as Confounding Mother*

Sally's cruel treatment of her first son continues to confound readers of *Peregrine Pickle.* A mischievous boy even at the young age of four, Perry was sent to a neighborhood day school to "be out of harm's way," which did little to deter his impish behavior.[74] Finding the schoolmistress at this school to be too lenient and ineffective in disciplining Perry, Sally dispatches him to a male pedagogue, whom she "ordered to administer such correction as the boy should in his opinion deserve," to the effect that he was "regularly flogged twice a day" for a year and a half. Capital punishment proved counterproductive, and the teacher declared Perry to be "the most obstinate, dull, and untoward genius that ever had fallen under his cultivation; instead of being reformed, he seemed rather hardened and confirmed in his vicious inclinations, and was dead to all sense of fear as well as shame" (53). "Extremely mortified at these symptoms of stupidity," Sally was advised to send

Perry to a boarding school, advice she "readily embraced" since she was pregnant with her second child, Gam, who "she hoped would console her for the disappointment she had met with in the unpromising talents of Perry" (54). When Perry's uncle Trunnion, also called the Commodore, returns home with the boy two years later, Sally "eyed [Perry] with tokens of affliction and surprise, and, bursting into tears, exclaimed her child was dead, and this was no other than an impostor whom they had brought to defraud her sorrow." Exiled from his home, Perry goes to live with Trunnion, who becomes his de facto parent thereafter (64). Sally continues to be unable to tolerate her son's presence and even forces her henpecked husband to reject Perry. By the novel's conclusion, Perry inherits both his father's and Trunnion's estates, without any reconciliation with his mother.

By all accounts, Sally exhibits characteristics of the unnatural mother in her treatment of Perry: unfeeling, unsympathetic, detached, absent, and allegedly murderous.[75] She sustains her "vicious aversion" of her son throughout the novel (64). Sally's rejection of her child, according to the maternal standards of the period, would be read as "monstrous," an abominable deviance from the norm. Francus notes that a mother's refusal to nurture her child "is the only available monstrosity available to the domesticated mother" because of the few choices she has. Maternal service determines a woman's virtue, with her power limited to her interactions with her children.[76] Nussbaum observes that the cult of motherhood, which reached its apex by midcentury, required that every woman across the globe capable of nurturing behavior, even those from the most "barbaric" and "savage" of cultures, conform to its standards.[77] Ever since the publication of Richard Allestree's *The Ladies Calling* (1673), the criteria for maternal conduct became a prevalent topic in conduct literature of the period, standards we still recognize and, to some degree, still expect today. Allestree's influential text meticulously outlined "the office and duty of a Mother," sketching what would become universal expectations for generations to follow: emotional tenderness toward her own children and diligent care and attendance throughout their childhood, including breastfeeding and early education.[78] By the middle of the eighteenth century, the state of motherhood became concomitant with moral and religious duty, and, as Toni Bowers notes, "mothering was increasingly imagined as a set of behaviors and attitudes entirely peculiar to women."[79] Ruth Perry observes maternal sentiment in literature as an "emotional force capable of moving a reading public."[80] So contrary is Sally's behavior to popular expectations of maternal feeling that it bewilders the men who witness it: Trunnion was "confounded," and her husband "so disconcerted and unsettled in his own belief . . . that he knew not how to behave towards the boy" (64).

While conduct manuals reinforced the naturalization of motherly love, evidence gestures to the philosophical skepticism regarding intuitive maternal feelings. Locke explicitly argues against innate principles and posits that mothering is a duty instilled by social expectations: "For, Parents preserve your Children, is so far from an innate Truth, that it is no Truth at all; it being a Command, and not a Proposition, and so not capable of Truth or Falshood."[81] The common consensus here is that a mother's fulfillment of her moral and social obligations toward her children—and, for Adam Smith, her nation—does not necessarily come from a biologically ingrained maternal instinct. The perfect mother in Allestree's vision is a production of gender discourse, a woman performing and enacting maternal identity in her social conditioning. Culture has become accustomed to watching this performance as natural, and Sally's character serves as a disruption to the maternal mythos.

### *The Mother's (Dis)Inheritance*

This examination of Sally's mothering is pertinent to the discussion of parental attribution because she appears to leave an indelible mark on her son, her temperament. Brian K. Nance's study of Sir Théodore Turquet de Mayerne, who served as the French King Henry IV's royal physician, shows de Mayerne considering the temperament of the patient's parents in the course of diagnosis and treatment.[82] In the following century, remnants of this practice remained; the physician William Buchan references Rousseau in his best-selling treatise *Domestic Medicine* (1769) for his argument that children do inherit their mother's constitutions: "An ingenious writer observes* [Rousseau], that on the constitution of mothers depends originally of that of their offspring."[83] While Buchan does not place sole responsibility on mothers, he nevertheless stresses the importance of mothers' obligation in educating themselves to properly care for their children, thereby contributing to and sustaining a healthy and productive society: "Did mothers know their importance, and lay it to heart, they would embrace every opportunity of informing themselves of the duties which they owe to their infant-offspring. It is theirs, not only to form the body, but also to give the mind its most early cast. They have it very much in their power to make men healthy or valetudinary, useful in life, or the bane of society."[84] The man-midwife John Maubray assigns the mother's habits of mind and body as the primary determinant of a child's temperament: "what Disorder soever of a vitious Nature derives itself this way from the mother, hath yet the greater Malignity, and more powerful Effect upon her Children; the Habits of her Body, Good or Bad, her Virtues or Vices, taking still a deeper root, or firmer Footing in the Constitution of the Foetus."[85] Smollett's focus on Sally's constitution and behavior during pregnancy becomes an essential factor in understanding Perry's character and promotes the negative parental attribution of the mother.

Despite Perry and his mother's limited time together, he bears her nature and inexplicable compulsion to inflict pain and ridicule. Sally's father, Mr. Appleby, enthusiastically consents to the marriage proposal and a swift wedding for his daughter, "to diffidence of his own daughter's complexion, which perhaps he thought too sanguine to keep much longer cool" (32). His belief that his daughter's "too sanguine" "complexion" requires release follows the medical account of bodily and psychological processes of the period. Building on Galen's theory that a healthy and virtuous body maintains balance and temperance, eighteenth-century hydraulic medical theory claimed that bodily temperance rested on the orderly circulation of the fluids and the regular discharge of excess material, thus maintaining the equilibrium of the hydraulic system.[86] The Dutch physician Jerome Gaub describes the sanguine person as "easily taught, ready, generous and flexible disposition, . . . coupled with negligence, want of foresight, inconstancy, immoderacy and an unbridled love of pleasure."[87] Sanguine persons suffer from an excess of animal spirits, according to Richard Blackmore: "The Passions and Appetites of these Men, from a redundancy of warm and lively Spirits, are more violent, and impatient of Restraint, than those in a cooler and less active Complexion," rendering them vulnerable to extreme swings of passion.[88] For example, Perry's erotic frustration with his beloved Emilia, at one point, becomes so dangerous that it necessitates bleeding to release the increasing pressure in his body. For sanguine people, like Sally and Perry, both emotional and physical health hinged on the constructive and temperate discharge of the powerful passions associated with their bodily temperament.

Thus, even before Perry's entrance in the novel, the stage is set for readers' expectations of him. The pregnant mother functions as a kind of narrative exordium, foreshadowing the child's propensities inherited from the mother's constitution. Beasley writes, "[Sally's] treatment of [Perry] may well be a reason why Perry behaves as he does. . . . Perry is all shallow compulsion and sparkling intelligence, fertile wit and active libido; he hardly changes at all through the novel."[89] Beasley takes this line of argument further by stating that "the boy is forced to grow up without any gentling restraints upon either his childhood rambunctiousness or, later, adolescent libido. Smollett never makes an issue of this deprivation in developing the character of his hero, but it does seem to have figured into his conception at least to some small extent; Perry's utter disregard for the selfhood of the women (including Emilia, until the very end) whose bodies he desires surely results in part from his lack of any model of the woman as feeling person."[90] While Perry's misogyny is evident, I am more inclined to agree with John Skinner that the narrative's structure is primarily dictated by the generic conventions of the ramble novel, rather than by character psychology.[91] Smollett's predecessors Rabelais, Cervantes, and Swift wrote novels disinterested in depth of character, some distance from the generic expectations of the realist and sentimental novels of Richardson. Simon Dickie observes that the ramble novels of the 1750s and 1760s like *Peregrine Pickle*, and *Tom Jones* before them, are full of "misogynist caricatures and unpleasant jokes about sexual violence" as "comic filler" to amuse their readers.[92]

At the risk of reading Perry's characterization anachronistically, I resist the urge to attribute Sally's cruelty and negligence of her firstborn son as the sole reason for shaping his character, despite the rich discourse of attributing the mother for the child's outcome, as I elaborated earlier in my reading of *Tristram Shandy*. We know that she was loving and affectionate toward her second son, Gam, who was born "rickety from the cradle," indicating that she is not entirely incapable of maternal warmth (79). Rather, I read Perry's unchecked coarseness and malice as an effect of homosocial bonds between men in the novel.

From Perry's childhood into adulthood, his companion Hatchway, his servant Pipes, and his friend Crabtree actively encourage and participate in playing pranks. Even the Commodore is amused by the young Perry's violent pranks on him. The intimacy among these men carries more authenticity and emotional weight than Perry's relationship with Emilia, who, like Sophia Western for Tom Jones, is meant to serve as the novel's moral center. Only she can regulate Perry's excess, with their marriage providing a neat and satisfactory closure to the rogue's reformation. And yet, *Peregrine Pickle* resists this conclusion. Perry remains incapable of restraint: He cajoles Emilia to marry quickly without her mother's attendance at the wedding, and he literally disengages Emilia's sister from an embrace so he can consummate their marriage without delay. Perry, now socially elevated with a virtuous wife and his father's and uncle's estates, makes a final circuit in town, where he pettily adopts "disdain" and "contempt" for members of the beau monde who had previously scorned him (780). Beasley's assessment is right in noting that Perry hardly evolves in the course of the novel, but his arrested development can be imputed beyond Sally's negligence. Smollett does draw on contemporaneous cultural and medical beliefs about the importance of how a child is brought into and up in the world, though it would be an oversimplification to solely attribute the mother for the son's attitudes toward women, especially when we consider the effect of homosocial relations on a male character's sensibility.

In contrast to Sally, Perry's father, Gamaliel Pickle, possesses an indifferent temperament, "little subject to refined sensations" and "scarce ever disturbed with violent emotions of any kind" (24). Governed by his temperamental wife, Gamaliel is cast as the dominated husband who "bore the yoke like an ox," without complaint. "This indolence, this sluggishness, this stagnation of temper, rendered Gamaliel incapable of withstanding arguments and importunity" (111). While Perry and Sally tend to instigate conflict, Gamaliel prefers to avoid any activity that requires mental, emotional, or physical exertion. The father's and son's contrasting temperaments would support the ovist perspective of preformation or the chance that he is not Perry's biological father. R. G. Collins proposes the possibility that Perry was conceived out of wedlock (which would also explain Mr. Appleby's swift consent to the marriage) to account for Sally's hatred and rejection of him.[93] Beasley admits that Perry's illegitimacy is "a kind of symbolic dispossession" that would justify his contemptible behavior but argues that Smollett abandons the possibility after the fourth chapter, that it "adds nothing in the way of depth to his hero's character."[94] My reading focuses more on Sally's reproductive contribution to Perry's character, offering a counterpoint to the masculinist embryological theories of the seventeenth and eighteenth centuries, without dismissing the possibility that his birth may be illegitimate.

### *Failure of Marriage as Cure (Again)*

If Mr. Appleby is implying that his daughter's passions need a sexual outlet for which marriage would be the remedy, her inability to temper her violent passions as a wife demonstrates the remedy's ineffectiveness. This treatment also fails to moderate her son's wild temperament. As McAllister has argued, Perry's fits of passion stem from his body's imbalance and its efforts to correct it through emotional discharge. Frustration from blocked erotic desire contributes to Perry's violence of mind; at one point, he raves like a "Bedlamite" for two hours after Emilia's rejection (409). In eighteenth-century medicine, marriage provided the erotic and emotional catharsis these young men so desperately needed: "Marriage offers a structure for emotional expression that is at once free and regulated, natural and rational. It represents the hygienic ideal of balance, of orderly yet free expression, in concrete form. . . . Marriage's rational pleasures simultaneously liberate and regulate desire."[95] This is explicitly true in *Roderick Random* (1748), Smollett's first, semiautobiographical novel published before *Peregrine Pickle*. In its conclusion, the newly wedded Roderick explains the regulating effects of marriage on himself: "The impetuous transports of my passion are now settled and mellowed into endearing fondness and tranquility of love, rooted by that intimate connexion and interchange of hearts, which nought but virtuous wedlock can produce."[96] Both novels follow a similar, rough trajectory of the comic romance culminating in the reformed young man's social elevation through fortune and marriage to a virtuous wife, but in contrast to Roderick's ultimate balancing of passion, Perry's emotional excess hardly calms. Born into affliction and tragedy, Roderick grows up with a true sense of injustice and alienation, from which his sensibility has been hardened by adversity. His mother died shortly after a traumatic delivery, violently induced by the emotional affliction from her father-in-law's rejection of her secret marriage. Roderick assumed that his father succumbed to grief and died by suicide shortly after, although he later discovers that his father is still alive and joyously reunites with him in Argentina. Perry, on the other hand, knew his parents but lives in the shadow of his mother's rejection and experiences no happy reconciliation with her in the end. Both mother and son petulantly grind their heels into the dirt. These two novels seem to suggest that it is not necessarily marriage but familial harmony that modulates the high energies of lost young men.

Similarly, marriage as a course of treatment fails to satisfy or regulate Sally's excess. Sexual temperance is demanded of the young woman from her maturity into adulthood. Unlike men, women did not have the same license to be sexual profligates, to give in to their erotic desires. Instead, women were expected to maintain strict bodily regulation to exhibit internal virtue. But, as I have shown in chapters 1 and 2, the medical community has consistently asserted that most women's bodies were inherently leaky and, as such, essentially incapable of bodily self-regulation. Mr. Appleby's belief that marriage would "cool" down his daughter reflects medicine's assertion of the potentially therapeutic nature of consistent, stable conjugal relations. *Peregrine Pickle*'s representation of sanguine persons regardless of sex demonstrates that passionate temperaments are incorrigible and that marriage as a course of corrective treatment is ineffective.

### *The Question of Women's Authority and Women's Knowledge*

As discussed earlier in this chapter, pregnancy was widely regarded as an intense and vulnerable state for both the mother and fetus. Since pregnant mothers' obstructed desires and irrational fears were believed to endanger their fetus, commentators supported the pregnant woman's rule in the household. Satirical works preceding *Peregrine Pickle* dramatized the pregnant woman taking full advantage of her privileged state in the household.[97] Smollett's representations of Sally's and Mrs. Grizzle's pregnancies ridicule the very notion that pregnant women be given free license out of the community's fear of harming the fetus. The cases of these two women challenge the mind-body models that explain the reciprocal processes of physiological and psychological motions. Sally feigns her cravings to humiliate her imposing sister-in-law, sending her on quests to escape her "teazing and disagreeable" company (39), while Mrs. Grizzle is convinced of her pregnancy (which turns out to be false) and subjects everyone, including her tragically credulous husband, to her whims and comical pretensions. Smollett's critique further extends to the ineptitude of professionally untrained midwives, which in turn, demonstrates his elitist attitudes regarding the superiority of degreed physicians like his friend and fellow Scotsman Smellie, who has been called "the master of British midwifery" and "the father of scientific obstetrics."[98] In *Peregrine Pickle*, women's ways of knowing are represented as foolish and potentially damaging to themselves.

### *Mrs. Grizzle/Trunnion and the Culture of Pregnancy*

For both pregnancy-centered episodes, Mrs. Grizzle is the butt of the joke, a frequent target of pranksters and tricksters, including her own sister-in-law.[99] When Mrs. Grizzle learns of Sally's pregnancy, she is determined to "exert her uttermost in nursing, tending, and cherishing" her, diligently studying popular works for midwifery, Nicholas Culpeper's *Directory for Midwives* (1651) and *Aristotle's Compleat and Experience'd Midwife* (1750?), and medical handbooks, the apothecary John

Quincy's *Pharmacopoeia* (1722) and Eliza Smith's *The Compleat Housewife* (1727). She rejects Sally's authority, reducing the mother's role to that of a vessel carrying "her brother's heir to light" (38). The narrative unequivocally demonstrates Sally's shamming of her pregnancy cravings as a ruse to escape her sister-in-law's oppressive surveillance. She invents onerous tasks for her sister-in-law with "ingenious craft" (43). Indeed, Sally is adept at assuming any disposition that would result in getting what she wants. Shortly after her marriage, Sally informs Mrs. Grizzle that she need no longer concern herself with household management: "This presumption was like a thunderbolt to Mrs. Grizzle, who began to perceive that she had not succeeded quite so well as she imagined, in selecting for her brother a gentle and obedient yoke-fellow, who would always treat her with that profound respect which she thought due to her superior genius, and be entirely regulated by her advice and direction" (37). Mrs. Grizzle had advocated for Sally's marriage to the indifferent Mr. Pickle so she could maintain her dominance over the household, only to discover that she had been duped. Jennifer Buckley writes, "Sally's conquest of Grizzle's domestic role is achieved with direct help of the trope of maternal longing."[100]

What follows is a comical representation of an anxious woman subjected to carrying out the whims of her pregnant sister-in-law to protect the Pickle heir. These requests included a pineapple, a fricassee of frogs from France, and strangely, to pinch her husband's ear and to pluck three black hairs from Trunnion's beard. Mrs. Grizzle's anxiety is brought on by her reading; the knowledge she acquires from these books informs her of the fragile and delicate state of pregnancy, cautioning how the mother's diet, behavior, environment, and temperament can significantly influence the outcome of the child. She does not question the sincerity of Sally's desires and is only driven to satisfy the pregnant mother's longings, no matter how "strangely diseased" she determines Sally's imagination has become (39). Mrs. Grizzle's character has already been established as a fool and a comic figure before these episodes, but her autodidactic efforts only amplify her foolishness. Perhaps it would have been better for all if she had never read these books, and in this way, Smollett illustrates a microcosmic moral panic regarding women's reading practices. Better to leave the complicated business of caring for pregnant women to trained professionals.

It is not insignificant that Smollett includes Culpeper's *Directory for Midwives* in Mrs. Grizzle's set of books. Culpeper was an untrained practitioner himself, thus serving as a poor instructor for his female readers in *Peregrine Pickle.* Although he practiced without a license, having only served as an apprentice to a London apothecary, Culpeper led a productive career in astrological medicine; he treated the poor, sometimes without a fee, and published eleven books in twenty editions before his death in 1654.[101] Culpeper advocated for democratizing the practice of medicine by teaching people, in popular vernacular rather than the abstruse and highly technical language of the highly educated, how to heal themselves with herbs found in their own gardens: "What an insufferable injury is it, That Men and Women should be trained up in such Ignorance, that when they are Sick and have Herbs in their Gardens conducing to their Cure, they are so Hoodwinked, that they know not their Vertues. Is not this to uphold a Company of Lazy Doctors, most of whose Covetousness out-weighs a Feather?"[102] He also knew that the College of Physicians, which he took to task for its power and corruption, would disapprove his pedagogical aim and method because instructing laypersons in the art of medicine would lead to ignorant and potentially dangerous practices. And yet, he insisted on sharing his knowledge of healing with the public, rather than hoarding it within a specialized circle of elite, degreed practitioners who charged exorbitant fees for their services. In *Directory for Midwives*, Culpeper explicitly discourages the use of a male midwife, who stands as an insult to the art of midwifery, as long as his directions are heeded correctly: "If you make use of them [my rules] you will find your work easie, and you need not call for the help of a Man-Midwife, which is a Disparagement, not only to your selves, but also to your Profession."[103] The fact that male midwives or physicians typically charged much higher fees than a woman midwife aligns with his antielitist views.

In Smollett's defense of William Smellie against the midwife Elizabeth Nihell's attack against male midwives, he champions the superiority of diagnosis based on experimental physiology and anatomy, training more readily available to men (though Smellie's lectures were open to midwives). While Smollett's critique is levied against professionally untrained midwives, it could easily apply to practitioners like Culpeper. In *The Critical Review,* Smollett sharply remarked, "The difference . . . between the male-practitioner who has attended lectures, and the female who has not, is this; the first understands the animal oeconomy, the structure of the human body, the cure of distempers, the art of surgery, together with the theory and practice of midwifery, learned from the observations of an experienced artist, and the advantage of repeated delivery: the last is totally ignorant of everything but what she may have heard from an ignorant nurse or midwife, or seen at the few labours she has attended."[104] Notably, Smollett's negative appraisal is for midwives who have not augmented their traditional hands-on training with formal education, such as studying Smellie's lectures. Traditionally, midwifery was a practiced skill taught from generation to generation without formal training.[105] Still, one can draw here that Smollett steadfastly believed in the superiority of degreed male practitioners in the art of midwifery. He wrote in *A Complete History of England* (1757) that "the art of Midwifery was elucidated by science, reduced to fixed principles, and almost wholly consigned into the hands of men practitioners."[106] Until the mid-eighteenth century, surgeons would be called to the delivery room only in cases of emergencies that required surgical intervention as a last resort. Later, more surgeons were asked to attend birthing women in normal deliveries.[107]

Smollett may be overstating the dominance of male midwives at the time he published *A Complete History of England*, but there is a possibility that half of deliveries were attended by male midwives by century's end.[108] His argument that the growing demand for male midwives stemmed from the public's recognition of their medical expertise over untrained midwives is an oversimplification of the cultural movement toward a higher value for science. Several factors contributed to this shift, including the decline of traditional midwifery licensing, the withdrawal of gentry midwives from practice out of social decorum, the view of village midwives as unsuitable guests in gentry households, and the increasing involvement of husbands, choosing male midwives from their social circles.[109]

By including Culpeper's *Directory for Midwives* as part of Mrs. Grizzle's collection, Smollett seems to extend his satire beyond the follies of reading women—their inability to read critically and/or lack of formal experience—to the authors whom they are reading. Most of *Peregrine Pickle*'s readers would recognize or even own these books. Through Mrs. Grizzle's humorous anxiety from following Culpeper's advice, readers could see the negative consequences of reading such material. In the 1790 edition of Smellie's *Treatise*, he himself refers to Culpeper's work "performances" that were "in great vogue with the midwives, and are still read by the lower sort, whose heads are weak enough for to admit such ridiculous notions."[110] At the same time, when we consider Culpeper's aims of dismantling the hierarchical structures of medical authority, which stood to profit handsomely from the uneducated, yet trusting, public, and his intentions for laypersons to take ownership over their own bodies and health, we find that Smollett might be writing from his own bias and experience, propagating the same kind of medical propaganda that devalued the skills of midwives written by male midwives in his time.

Stark differences are evident in the style and content of Culpeper's and Smellie's books. Smellie's volumes are a straightforward collection of cases with prescriptions based on his and others' experience in the practice of midwifery and anatomy, intended for a professional audience. Culpeper's books read like primers with a glossary for uninformed laypersons, and he frequently makes digressions into political allusions and commentaries that protested the general abuses of power.[111] Culpeper is more confident, calling his prescriptions and advice as "cures" (the word occurs 124 times in *Directory for Midwives*), while Smellie is more cautious to promote a particular treatment as such. There is much more emphasis on the salubrious influence of humoral nonnaturals in Culpeper's work, which is perhaps why diet figures largely in successful conceptions and births. These differences could be attributed to each practitioner's training (or lack thereof). Culpeper categorically argues that parents' poor diet and exercise are the "two general Evils" attributed to the "chief cause of Death of Children in their Infancy."[112] Smellie, on the other hand, attributes most unnecessary maternal and infant deaths to practitioners' mishandling of specific cases.

Culpeper's cautionary tone and alarming language would inevitably create unnecessary anxiety and distress for his readers, as illustrated in Smollett's characterization of Mrs. Grizzle. A single poor choice, from conception to birth, could produce a dead or monstrous child. Culpeper warns pregnant women from "sharp meats, very bitter or salt, and things that can provoke terms, as garlic, onions, olives, mustard, fennel, and all spices. . . . Summer fruits are nought for her."[113] Heeding this advice, Mrs. Grizzle puts Sally on a heavily restricted diet based on the advice from reading materials that warned about the abortive effects of certain fruits and vegetables. When Sally intended to eat a peach, a summer fruit Culpeper forbids pregnant women from consuming, Mrs. Grizzle "fell on her knees in the garden, entreating her, with tears in her eyes, to desist such a pernicious appetite." Sally complies, but then Mrs. Grizzle recalls that if "her sister's longing was balked, the child might be affected with some disagreeable mark or deplorable disease" (38). For Culpeper, pregnancy cravings, which are a natural consequence of what the mother needs to nourish her child, could lead to miscarriage if left unsatisfied: "If the Body of the Woman be thus disturbed, of Necessity the Child within her must be disturbed also; therefore Nature as the chief Artificer calls for such food a must make fitting Blood for the nourishment or increase of the Child. Your Child is nourished by your own Blood, your Blood is bread by your diet, rectified or marred by your exercise, idleness, sleep or watching, etc."[114] Mrs. Grizzle begs Sally to eat the fruit and then forcibly administers a cordial she prepared as "an antidote to the poison she had received" (38). Confused about the right course of action, Mrs. Grizzle desperately follows both approaches and hopes for the best, demonstrating the contradictions in Culpeper's advice.

This brings us to the question of the pineapple, the recently fashionable and exotic fruit Sally longs for, claiming to have dreamt of eating it. Mrs. Grizzle searches "through the whole country for this unlucky fruit" for three days, "unmindful of her health, and careless of her reputation" (41). G. S. Rousseau points out that the pineapple's danger for pregnant women was a prevailing opinion at the time, citing several medical texts and dictionaries to support this claim.[115] Collins, then, uses this popular belief as possible proof of Sally's intent to abort her fetus, although it is not clear whether she had actually eaten the fruit once Mrs. Grizzle acquired it for her, which casts doubt on her abortive intent. The passage Rousseau cites from Culpepper is actually found in his other book, *The English Physician* (1725), in which he warns women of the abortive effects of pineapples: "It marvelously helpeth all the Diseases of the Mother used inwardly, or applied outwardly, procuring Women's Courses, and expelling the dead Child and After-birth, yea, it is so powerful upon those Feminine parts that it is utterly forbidden for Women with Child, and that it will cause abortment or delivery before the time. . . . Let Women forbear it if they be with Child, for it works violently upon the Feminine Part."[116] Rousseau's reference to Culpeper begs the question of how seriously Smollett took his views, considering the novelist's medical training and his support for Smellie. Smollett seems to have drawn from popular notions about the abortive effects of pineapples only to ridicule the convictions of pseudomedical experts like Culpeper and the people who believe them.

Indefatigable about protecting Sally's fetus and susceptible to the alarmist rhetoric of Culpeper, Mrs. Grizzle behaves in extremes. Upon hearing Sally's desire for a pineapple, Mrs. Grizzle screams and embraces her sister "with a sort of hysterical laugh, importing horror rather than delight" (39). Then, for three days and nights, she canvasses the whole county for the desired pineapple in a mania. She faints upon hearing that no pineapples can be found and later falls into a "violent fever" from the enterprise. Her frenzy to satisfy Sally's desires leaves her vulnerable to her neighbors' ruses to profit from her desperation. Informed by a gardener that pineapples were in short supply, she happily pays five guineas for a few, unaware that there were still a hundred left. Represented as the fool with limited self-possession and intellectual discernment, Mrs. Grizzle, by her leaky femaleness, heightens Smollett's caricature of the amateur layperson tinkering in serious medical subjects by deploying it in a body incapable of serious and, by default, masculine restraint.

## *Mrs. Trunnion's Mole and the Trauma of Disappointment*

Mrs. Grizzle, who later becomes Mrs. Trunnion upon her marriage to the retired, curmudgeonly naval officer, undeniably fits the model of the gullible fool. Through her experience, the satire mostly targets the culture of pregnancy that generates unnecessary panic and relies on the experiential knowledge of women. This portrayal parallels Smollett's treatment of Tabitha Bramble's enthusiastic (albeit short-lived) Methodism in *Humphry Clinker*, in which he also satirizes the immoderate passions of women. Shortly after Mrs. Trunnion's wedding, she experiences a false pregnancy, withdrawing from society and turning to drink in secret. The aftermath of this traumatic event, in which Mrs. Grizzle finds succor in substance abuse, demonstrates the enduring and tragic consequence of dangerous and willful ignorance.

Early in the novel, Smollett signals Mrs. Trunnion's incapability of reproduction, and this inability becomes a source of humor. Though she is only thirty, her name suggests maturity. In Hogarthian caricature of her physiognomy and figure, the language of humoralism portrays her as a grotesque and possibly barren woman: "Exclusive of a very wan (not to call it sallow) complexion, which, perhaps, was the effects of her virginity and mortification, she had a cast in her eyes that was not at all engaging; and such an extent of mouth, as no art or affectation could contract into any proportionable dimension" (24). In humoralism, women become drier as they age. The physician John Freind explains, "For as old age creeps on, the humours every day become both less redundant, and the fibres of the vessels grow more rigid and hard. . . . Elderly women are more dry and abound less with blood."[117] For modern readers, Mrs. Trunnion at thirty is hardly at the age when women cannot become pregnant, but in this period, young women were cautioned not to wait too long to get married. In *Aristotle's Masterpiece*, a woman's value tied to her virginity has an expiration date: "if they keep [their virginity] too long, it grows useless, or at least loses much of its Value: a stale Virgin (if such a Thing there be) being look'd upon like an old Almanack out of Date."[118] Her virginity at this age could also lead to a state of "mortification," which may mean a state of embarrassment or, in the medical world, the death of a body part or necrosis. Her presumably late entry into marital life could not possibly produce a viable fetus since her reproductive system has *died* from celibacy as a single woman, in addition to the increasingly inflexibility of her "fibers," crucial in regulating menses and gestation. For John Maubray, her womb's "mortified" state engenders a "mole" caused by an "imperfect conception" from an "infirmity of the forming faculty" of imbalanced menstrual blood.[119] Like Walter, though he is much older than Mrs. Grizzle when he conceived Tristram with his wife, advanced age worked against true (or healthy) conception. Mrs. Grizzle's dry and hollow body becomes the stage for a morality play, with the wishful woman severely punished for the hubris in her own bodily epistemology.

Smollett continues his satire on pregnancy culture with Mrs. Trunnion's false pregnancy, but to a different degree. Since she was never pregnant, her afflictions and her desires can only be attributed to being purely psychosomatic, thus refuting the idea that the community should rely on the pregnant woman's account. Early modern medical texts and midwifery manuals were reluctant to definitively confirm pregnancy because it was difficult to determine with certainty that a woman was with child. The signs of conception, such as dimness of eyes, pall complexion, and fatigue, could easily be mistaken as symptoms of other diseases.[120] Even cessation of the menses could signify pregnancy or the presence of an abnormal uterine growth, commonly termed a "mole." Until the parents held a living, breathing infant in their arms, it was nearly impossible to determine if the woman carried a child or a "foul mass of flesh that comes to no perfection."[121] Mrs. Trunnion mistakenly assumes her body to exhibit symptoms of pregnancy, such as faintness, vomiting, hardened breasts, and a prominent stomach (63), when, in all likelihood, a mole resided in her womb. Unsurprisingly, the community did not question Mrs. Trunnion's claims. She is, after all, a married woman who presumably enjoyed conjugal pleasures. In addition, as far back as *Aristotle's Masterpiece*, most people maintained that the mother herself apprehended pregnancy even before the cessation of her menses.[122] Smollett, then, challenges the long-standing notion of women's experiential knowledge as an accurate way of determining pregnancy.

Like Sally, Mrs. Trunnion relishes her newfound power, and her behavior becomes the setup of the long, cruel joke: "She knew this was the proper season for vindicating her own sovereignty, and accordingly employed the means which nature had put in her power. There was not a rare piece of furniture or apparel for which she did not long; and one day, as she went to church, seeing Lady Stately's equipage arrive, she suddenly fainted away" (63). She played the part of a pregnant woman in public: "In all her visits and parties she seized every opportunity of declaring her present condition, observing that she was forbid by her physicians to taste such a pickle, and that such a dish was poison to a woman in her way; nay, where she was on a footing of familiarity, she affected to make wry faces, and complained that the young rogue began to be very unruly, writhing herself into divers contortions, as if she had been grievously incommoded by the mettle of this future Trunnion" (64). She carried on thus, and her husband's vanity indulged in the same fantasy, purchasing whatever extravagance she desired and imagining a life at sea for the boy (63, 64). While the community could not directly experience her pregnancy, Mrs. Trunnion sought to communicate her body's affliction through oral and physical performance, giving authenticity to what she imagined was real gravidity. The melodramatic performance increases the comic irony of the joke; the higher she rises on the pedestal of pregnancy, the harder the joke lands, with her barrenness revealed.

While Mrs. Trunnion is the satirical target, Smollett partly attributes the Trunnions' becoming "the standing joke of the parish" (65) to the incompetence of midwives. In a series of false alarms when Mrs. Trunnion believes she is in the throes of labor and her seemingly pregnant body becomes less apparent ("she was sensibly diminished in the waist . . . a reduction of Mrs. Trunnion as might have been expected after the birth of a full-grown child"), the midwives continue to "feed Mrs Trunnion with hopes of a speedy and safe delivery" (65). Even after the male midwife declares that she had never been pregnant, the Trunnions and the midwives carry on the charade for three weeks until she appeared "as lank as a greyhound, and they were furnished with other unquestionable proofs of their having been deceived" (65). The couple then withdraw to themselves in a "paroxysm of shame and confusion" (65). The medical consensus surrounding the possibility of this event is the suppression of the wife's menses. Jean Astruc claims three cases when the patient was suspected of being with child from the swollen belly and the absence of the menses, but it was the retention of menstrual blood in the womb that caused the swelling.[123] The midwives, perhaps for the promise of a reward after the successful and healthy delivery of a wealthy mother, fueled the "sweet delusion" of pregnancy. However, the couple's hopes of an heir deflated just as quickly as Mrs. Trunnion's belly.

Through this episode, Smollett engages in the male midwife and female midwife debate in the period, asserting the professional ineptitude and medical ignorance of women without formal training in the obstetric sciences.[124] This criticism anticipates the silencing of the female voice in the nineteenth century, when medical authority did not rely on the pregnant woman's experiential knowledge, and perhaps even dismissed or doubted it, to gain more knowledge about obstetric science.[125] This mistake had permanent consequences for the once-optimistic couple: The would-be mother lives in alcohol-soaked seclusion, and the husband continues to be haunted by the shadow of the quondam possibility of issue. While Smollett satirizes the woman's ability to know her body for comic effect, the bleak representation of the Trunnions' response to the mole is undeniably tragic.

While both Mr. and Mrs. Trunnion endured the disappointment of this ordeal, the wife indubitably sustains a longer-term emotional response to this trauma. The Commodore "in a little time weathered his disgrace" but made it "his chief aim . . . to be absent from his own house as much as possible" to avoid the "souring" of his wife's temper (51). Mrs. Trunnion was bedridden in anguish for weeks, and even when she was able to join society again, "her misfortune had made such an impression on her mind, that she could not bear the sight of a child, and trembled whenever conversation happened to turn upon a christening" (51). Through the ordinary sights and sounds of her community, she relives her trauma over and over again, mourning the loss of her reproductive story.

Unlike the happily coupled Tabitha Bramble and Captain Obadiah Lismahago of *Humphry Clinker*, whom Jason Farr views as a positive articulation of "the resistance to reproductive futures by imagining marriage as accessible to those in their advanced years," the Trunnions have so deeply invested in the discourse of reproductive futurism that the loss of what they had imagined as an issue has damaged their relationship beyond repair.[126] And for Mrs. Trunnion, this damage fractures her sense of self: How could she know who she is or why she is if she does not know her own body? Gélis harshly remarks that in the cultural view at the time, "a barren couple was an aberration; they might as well be dead already, since they had no future." It is the barren woman herself who betrays nature, however: "By failing in her duty and breaking the continuity of the family she is damaging the very work of creation."[127] While Mrs. Trunnion's pregnant pageantry and ignorant insistence can be read as a broad satiric and misogynistic vignette on the foolishness of women, the extent to which her trauma has taken root into her consciousness and selfhood evokes the reader's sympathies, especially when considering Smollett's generally flat treatment of women in *Peregrine Pickle.*

### *The Disappearance of the Pregnant Woman*

The paradox that emerges here is that the more medical attention is being paid to the female body, the more absent she becomes. In the sixteenth and seventeenth centuries, the word for "to give birth" in French textbooks is *s'accoucher*, a reflexive verb signifying the woman's active role. A century later, the increasing intervention of the male obstetrician removed her involvement, reflected in the use of *accoucher* or the passive *etre accouchee.*[128] Ernelle Fife compares the chronicles of birth between female midwives and male obstetricians, noting that physicians' "texts eliminate the women's story and replace it with the clinical tale told from a male perspective."[129] Female midwives preferred to refer to the mother as "woman" rather than "patient," identifying women as active subjects.[130] In contrast, male midwives treated the woman as an object of the narrative and ended case histories with an autopsy, leaving students of obstetrics to imagine the woman merely as a body. As male physicians' writing became more clinical and scientific, women's stories were eliminated.[131] Fife writes, "If the male midwives' chosen discourse reflects their medical practice, then women lost a compassionate medical care-giver. Their discourses do seem to replace empathy with scientific professionalism. If the male midwives' language communicates their attitudes, then as the art of midwifery developed into the medical science of obstetrics, patients became physical objects to be manipulated, not women with stories to be heard."[132] Gélis notes the same change, that obstetric expertise took precedence over women's experiential knowledge and removed empathy: "It is only exceptionally that the sufferings of mother and child are mentioned at all."[133]

With the proliferation of male midwives, the once-secret arena of obstetric knowledge between women became public, both in medicine and in popular culture. These men enjoyed a kind of celebrity status through public lectures, which included presentations of nude female bodies, and their publicly lauded involvement with establishing philanthropic maternity hospitals.[134] Cody writes, "By the early 1800s, these men had a very broad and widely accepted authority over all aspects related to sex and reproduction, as they claimed not only to unveil the secret world of reproduction, but to improve upon its possibilities, for instance, by curing disorders related to menstruation or saving vulnerable neonates."[135] Moreover, male midwives actively campaigned to discredit female midwives. They argued with Nihell that sharing the same sex with their female patients does not necessarily make female midwives better practitioners. Louis LaPeyre emptied the female midwife of her femininity and humanity, calling her an "animal with nothing of the woman left," whereas the male midwife has a "tender and humane disposition . . . endowed with sensibility of soul," able to "sympathyze with the evils and afflictions which human nature is liable to," and "extremely compassionate, especially with regard to the pain [of women]."[136] Not content to merely seize the means of reproduction, male midwives sought to demolish the credibility of community-based female experiential knowledge en masse.

## CONCLUSION

As an active site of creation, the maternal body pulsated with latent political, scientific, and domestic power in the eighteenth century. A realm inaccessible to male experience and knowledge, pregnancy and birth were women's dominions. Husbands literally waited outside as the woman midwife, mother, and other women in the birth circle brought new life to the world in a private and sacred space. The state of pregnancy provided women temporary power over their households, their bodies, and their men. While medical knowledge on animal generation advanced considerably in the era with William Harvey's *de Generatione*, the science of human conception and generation remained a mystery, prompting physicians to speculate on the subject. These speculations from animalculists and ovists alike maintained gender hierarchies in medicine, attributing primacy of healthy generation to the father, who either implanted a miniature version of himself in the womb or provided the soul that activated the menstrual mass into human shape. Medical discourse, through the generation and maternal impressions debates, needed to confirm the father's sovereignty to reinforce patrilineal structures of political power. As comic novels, both *Tristram Shandy* and *Peregrine Pickle* target the long tradition of female dominance in midwifery in the context of the emerging, professional, and male-dominated branch of obstetrics.

Walter Shandy's comic frustration with the women in *Tristram Shandy* stems from his desire to control conception and birth, to claim responsibility for the fetus's outcome even at the cost of embodying a frail and fragile masculinity. The father's role in true birth was concentrated at the time of conception, yet the mother was held responsible for fetal development, delivery, and the child's future physical and mental well-being. Tristram's eventual misfortunes and physical frailty are primarily attributed to his mother's "unseasonable question" during coitus, which distracted Walter from doing the job properly. Walter believes that his advanced age and decreased vitality worked against the production of a healthy baby, so he turns to policing his wife's behavior and care of herself. If Mrs. Shandy does not avoid mental and emotional disturbance while pregnant, she could potentially exacerbate the weakened state of the fetus. Existing maternal impressions debates and prevailing medical attitudes about essential female physical and emotional frailty increased the urgency to a social and moral imperative. Excess passion could potentially cause miscarriage or fetal deformity, so the pregnant woman must be kept calm. Even though hysteria treatment strongly recommended marriage and motherhood as a way of controlling symptoms, practitioners believed that pregnant women had even more difficulty managing their emotions. What is more, if the pregnant woman did not give vent to her emotions, this obstruction of passions could only harm herself and the fetus she carried. All of these contradictory beliefs arrived at the same place: possessing a woman's body. Mrs. Shandy could not help Tristram recover from his injuries incurred at conception. Maternal attribution in fetal and subject formation could only be granted in the production of an unhealthy child.

Despite Walter's efforts for reproductive control, the women in *Tristram Shandy* refuse to cede their authority, trusting their own expertise in pregnancy and midwifery as an exclusively female arena of knowledge. The lack of women's direct experience—especially Mrs. Shandy's labor—implies a begrudging recognition of women's bodily agency and authority. The communal quality of labor and birth temporarily elevates female dominance in the household, much to Walter's resentment. However, this brief reprieve from male surveillance and policing, long in practice for hundreds of years, is now threatened by the encroachment of emerging obstetric ideas. Though Walter's efforts are comically unsuccessful, especially in convincing his wife to undertake a caesarean birth, they presage the weakening of women's dominion in the practice of midwifery.

*Peregrine Pickle* also engages with the parental attribution debates, but with a more definite vision of negative maternal influence on the child's outcome. Perry seems to have wholly inherited Sally's sanguine temperament, with the monstrous mother passing on her appetite for cruelty to her son. Smollett's inclusion of Sally's behavior in exploiting the culture of pregnancy serves as a kind of narrative exordium, meant to signal Perry's likeness to his mother, and promotes the same belief of negative maternal attribution debated in *Tristram Shandy*. However, I have explained that laying the blame for Perry's unchecked personality at Sally's feet is an oversimplification; homosocial relations between men can also shape a young man's character. Smollett may hold the humoral belief that nothing can change one's temperament, but temperament alone does not determine one's complexion.

And on the validity and reliability of women's bodily authority over pregnancy, labor, and birth, Smollett's sharper satire mocks the laywomen and female midwives who assert more expertise over degreed male midwives. Unlike the near absence of women's direct experience in *Tristram Shandy*, *Peregrine Pickle* centers Sally and Mrs. Trunnion in these early episodes as subjects of comic irony. Mrs. Trunnion is especially the target of several jokes as the misinformed and anxious female reader of Culpeper's *Directory for Midwives* and as the desperately hopeful prey of avaricious and ignorant women midwives. Neither the community nor the women midwives question the truth of Mrs. Trunnion's pregnancy, and this total trust on the woman's experience ends tragically with the enduring trauma of loss. While Smollett's biting satire concentrates on the foolishness of women, he sympathetically represents Mrs. Trunnion's suffering in grief.

If marriage and motherhood, as proposed by medical and social models at the time, promised to fix women's biological ailments resulting from their essential "leakiness" and excess, *Tristram Shandy* and *Peregrine Pickle* demonstrate the reproductive anxieties that undermine the effectiveness of this cure. Walter claims that he cannot control his wife, Sally's marriage fails to cool her sanguine temperament, and Mrs. Trunnion is left disappointed and humiliated in her childlessness. And if the comic novel conventionally closes with the reconciliation of family to reestablish domestic harmony, both novels defy this neat resolution. The Shandy household is gathered together in the final pages of the novel, but the story ends with bickering. And in *Peregrine Pickle*, which I read as more cynical than

*Tristram Shandy*, mother and son continue to be estranged, with Perry hardly changing into an honorable and dignified gentleman in his married state. Marriage has not "fixed" anyone or anything. These comic representations of women's experience of pregnancy and birth after marriage dramatize another, less palatable reality of life after the wedding, a litmus test of the effectiveness of marriage as a cure. In the debates on parental attribution, maternal impressions, and midwifery, women are yet again blamed for their own, their children's, and their family's misfortunes. Ultimately, these tensions were quieted in the years to come in the age of clinical medicine and the age of Victorian motherhood. A negative correlation of female power emerged: As women lost control over their own pregnancies and births from male interventions in obstetrics, their ability to mother was heralded as the highest point of femininity.

Chapter 4 turns to Charlotte Lennox's *The Female Quixote*, and I align the discourses of women's nervous, hysterical embodiment in *Joseph Andrews* and *Tom Jones* with the affective experience of women's reading practices begun in my discussion of *Peregrine Pickle*. As I mentioned in the introduction, *The Female Quixote* is a long rape joke; Arabella's unrelenting fear of male sexual violence, learned through her mother's French romances, is the basis of much of the novel's humor. Arabella's community dismisses her feelings of terror as madness, and yet again, the woman's authority of knowing herself and her own emotional embodiment is questioned.

4

# ROMANTIC (MIS)READINGS AND NERVOUS SYMPATHY IN CHARLOTTE LENNOX'S *THE FEMALE QUIXOTE* (1752)

IN THE LONG EIGHTEENTH CENTURY, the relationship between bodies and books was a vexed one. Critics of the novel worried over the moral impact of reading, especially in the ways in which women, with their impressionable minds and bodies, were susceptible to the corrupting nature of the novel's immoral story lines. Medical practitioners contributed to these debates by theorizing how certain reading practices could be understood as a medical problem. Recreation, including reading, was an important consideration in maintaining good health as an external influence on the body. Eighteenth-century medicine still relied on the Galenic doctrines of the nonnaturals, how external factors influence emotion, thus causing physical symptoms and illness. The physician George Cheyne, who specialized in nervous disease, wrote in his *Essay on Health and Long Life* (1724) that "the passions have a greater influence on health, than most people are aware of."[1] The idea that the practice of reading is a form of external stimulation suggests a medical component to a person's emotional state. In my previous discussion on hysteria in chapter 2, women were imagined to have finer sensibilities, making them more vulnerable to physiological and emotional imbalances through their contact with other people, places, and things. Women's interaction with books, then, was a critical part of the conversation regarding the maintenance of good health.

In this chapter, I continue the discussion begun in my readings on Fielding's *Joseph Andrews* and *Tom Jones* and women's nervous embodiment with Charlotte Lennox's *The Female Quixote* (1752) and the affective experience of women's reading. In *The Female Quixote*, Arabella, a young woman who lives a sheltered life in her father's castle, nourishes her mind and imagination with her dead mother's "Store of [badly translated French] Romances."[2] The novel's humor primarily hinges on a comedy of incongruity: Arabella's exacting code of conduct, derived directly from the gendered models of virtue in these romances, makes her appear as a comic absurdity to others, including her suitor and cousin, Mr. Glanville. Their prevailing judgment often attributes her strange behavior to some form of mental pathology resulting from her intensive reading practices. However, between these fits of "Phrenzy," she is described as a young woman of "fine sense," praised "to the skies for [her] wit" (60, 61). Her family and acquaintances find it challenging to reconcile these two sides of Arabella, especially with her emotional responses to what they believe to be imaginary dangers. Unlike the delusional and elderly Don Quixote, whom the novel parodies, Arabella does not mistake windmills for monsters; instead, she uses her learning gleaned from her mother's library and her keen senses to suspect any man as a potential rapist. Arabella's emotional responses, like many other eighteenth-century novel heroines, underscore her social inexperience. But what sets her apart is her unwavering and absolute certainty of how the world is ordered through the moral education she received from reading romances—a world in which women must do everything within their power to avoid male tyranny and sexual violence.

I argue that Arabella's moral education acquired from her mother's books equipped her with the foresight to protect herself from the very real dangers of male predation. As a young, inexperienced woman of noble birth, she identified with the heroines in these romances and read how their sex and station rendered them especially vulnerable to male violence. These narratives functioned like conduct books, giving Arabella guidance on how to avoid or escape potentially harmful situations. The process of rereading these books developed a reflexive response in Arabella to such situations, in which her mind and body acted in vitalist sympathy together in self-direction and self-preservation. Vitalism is a monistic system of physiology that rejects the dualist Cartesian paradigm in which the mind operates independently of the body. Instead, vitalist epistemology relied on the body's absolute sympathy with each of its parts, with the "spirit" in the brain and the heart acting in a circle. For most of the people around Arabella, she speaks and behaves confusingly, but if we assess her behavior by the principles of empiricism, she is rational and perceptive: She trusts her own bodily senses and reasoning, and most of the time, as I will show, her fears of predation are justified, enabling her to avoid harm from male violence. Vitalist medical theory helps explain the discrepancy between Arabella's superior wit and apparent madness seeded by her moral education from romances, that her genuine emotional and physical responses to perceived threats to her autonomy are expressions of the operations of nervous sympathy. To put it simply, in Arabella's case, the practice of reading seems to train her nerves.

Critics have interpreted Lennox's second novel, *The Female Quixote*, as a work that primarily demonstrates women's contentious relationship to the romance.[3] Margaret Ann Doody observes that by the middle of the century, romance was passé, "and with it women's whole literary experience for two generations."[4] *The Female Quixote* exhibits the tensions between the diminishing popularity of romances and the emerging ethos of Augustan satire and between feminine and masculine perceptions and experience. While the novel uses the romantic form to differentiate itself, as Laurie Langbauer suggests, the generic disparity between the two ultimately dissolves, subverting that demarcation: "*The Female Quixote* both mocks and lauds its heroine's quixotism, and the way it ridicules romance actually exposes the attractions of that form. What it locates as romance's problems—the disorder and rigidity of its form, the ambiguities of its language—become its own."[5] These distinctions are directly related to gender; the novel associates the dangers of romance with female transgressions. The problems of irrationality, silliness, and unruliness of romance, Langbauer asserts, are also the problems linked with women.[6] And most recently, Amelia Dale asserts that representations of impressionable quixotic figures were entangled with the period's anxieties around gender and subjectivity.[7]

Arabella's unintelligibility at times is characterized as fits of madness, incongruous with her other idealized feminine traits of "great sensibility and softness" (*Female Quixote*, 15). Langbauer identifies this apparent madness as a metaphor of pathology for the romance: "Arabella's excesses of behavior actually reflect what is wrong with romance. . . . Through her, *The Female Quixote* shows that romance is excessive fiction, so excessive that it is nonsensical, ultimately mad."[8] Critics have considered Arabella's "mad romancing" as living out a fantasy of female power subjugated by patriarchal dominance and have admired her character for giving expression to the desire for empowerment that had long been suppressed. Langbauer contends that romance is "empowering, not imprisoning," and "the conventions of romance are what might give women voice."[9] To everyone's discomfort, Arabella gives voice to the sexual violence to which women are always vulnerable. By repeatedly insisting on the possibility of rape, she directs attention to herself as a sexual object and to any man as a potential rapist. Wendy Motooka argues that "Quixotism is not incomprehensible lunacy, but a trope to disparage those who adhere to a different set of political values, supported by a different political rationale."[10] The books in her library may be "senseless fictions," but the historical truth of women's victimization at the hands of male violence is real.[11] Arabella's quixotism empties the father and the husband of their roles as affectionate protectors in the paternalist model and imbues them with patriarchal terror instead.

The moral precepts Arabella has learned from these histories direct her imagination and behavior, which ultimately must be reformed for the sake of pacifying masculine anxiety. Only the men in *The Female Quixote* are the most distressed by her strict adherence to a moral code that brings embarrassment to her family. Arabella's mother educates her daughter from the grave through her library of romances, the final legacy for her only child. Forced into seclusion from society by her husband, the Marchioness purchased these books to "soften a Solitude which she found very disagreeable" (7). Arabella's resistance to her father, the Marquis, and to Glanville (as the next man who seeks to dominate her) resurrects and fulfills her mother's inner yearnings for freedom from an unpleasant life of patriarchal subjugation. Debra Malina observes, "The romances stand as both evidence and emblem of the repression of the mother: the actual mother bought and read them because the patriarch did not allow her to engage in activities she might have preferred, and the same patriarch wishes to destroy them because the women's fantasies they contain 'turn' the minds of young women, rendering them uncontrollable. In her reading of them, then, Arabella has already performed a political act of recovering and allying herself with the absent mother in defiance of the father."[12] Both mother and daughter are subjected to the tradition of victimization as a consequence of masculine anxiety and humiliation, for the Marquis's banishment and disgrace from court society, a metaphoric castration of political power, forced him to "devote the rest of his Life to Solitude and Privacy" (5). Glanville will ultimately perpetuate this pattern in removing the mortification in his life at the cost of Arabella's identity.

As the focus of the final chapter and the only novel I examine written by a woman, *The Female Quixote* subverts the fundamental essentialism of the medical theories explored so far in this book. The pervasive medical belief that runs through theories of menstruation, hysteria, and pregnancy asserts that women are physically incapable of self-regulation. This principle, as I have demonstrated, mutually reinforces the moral and cultural imperative for the patriarchal policing of women. Lennox turns the justification for this control on its head by angling the camera on the ways in which men themselves are actually the ones incapable of managing their passions. The men in Arabella's life, whose prescribed roles are to love and protect her, threaten her with violence and imprisonment to break her intractability. Her willfulness is the killjoy of everyone's happiness, to use Sara Ahmed's definition, and Arabella disrupts the liberal realism that relies on the fantasy of a peaceful heterosexual patriarchy by exposing the existing joyless social order.[13] Regina Barreca notes that this disruption is a recurring theme in women's comic writing: "Much of women's comic play has to do with power and its systematic misappropriation. Women's humor is about our reclamation of certain forms of control over our own lives. Humor allows us to gain perspective by ridiculing the implicit insanities of patriarchal culture."[14] *The Female Quixote*'s comic ironies of men in excess are certainly radical, but women humorists can make these representations more palatable to audiences.[15] This was certainly the case, if we measure this palatability with the novel's broad success with male readers such as Samuel Johnson. Still, Lennox ridicules an unjust social system against women: If comedy is mapped and marked by the author's subjectivity, Lennox's creation of Arabella's willfulness reflects her own anger as a professional woman writer in a deeply gendered world. Barreca continues, "Comedy resembles anger: it is channeled through pathways not blocked by fear and authority and is therefore often misdirected. Often it turns directly against the self as the simplest target. Women's comedy is marginal, liminal, concerned with and defined by its very exclusion from convention, by its aspects of refusal and its alliance with subversive feminine symbols. The difference of women is viewed as a risk to culture."[16] Comedy is the vehicle to illustrate the absurdities of the world, and for Barreca, "Women's comedy functions along such lines because it underscores the way women's narratives often depend on the split between the 'real' and the 'imaginary,' the incongruity between women's experience and so-called universal experience, the disparity between what women know to be true and what they are told is the truth."[17] Arabella's "madness" in refuting the systemic myths of patriarchy is both willful and prescient, and her nervous sympathy, developed through years of "bad reading," authentically reflects her terror of victimization from masculine violence.

## WOMEN'S READING PRACTICES AND "LOOSE AND WANDERING IMAGINATIONS"

*The Female Quixote* can be interpreted as a case study of women's reading practices as both an intellectual and affective experience in which ideas become imprinted onto the physical body. Arabella's ideas about life were shaped by the content in the books she regarded as true histories, ideas woven into the fabric of her mind and body. The Marquis restricts the young Arabella, keeping her in confinement in his castle and taking sole responsibility for her education. Her early "fondness for reading . . . extremely delighted the Marquis," and he allowed her free use of his library, which included her late mother's poorly translated romances (7). From this course of study, "Her ideas, from the manner of her life, and the objects around her, had taken a romantic turn; and supposing Romances were real pictures of life, from them she drew all her notions and expectations. By them she was taught to believe, that love was the ruling principle of the world; that every other passion was subordinate to this; and that it caused all the happiness and miseries of life" (7). Solitary, extensive, and passive reading of romances was believed to be particularly harmful to an inexperienced young woman since it presumably instilled false, yet indelible, ideas about how the world works. Though the Marquis was initially delighted by Arabella's intense consumption of books, they become the source of her filial disobedience. The cultural and medical discourse insisted on the appropriate way women should read, which could only be in compliance with their subjugated roles as daughters and wives. Arabella's refusal to conform is read as madness, but she sees the world as it truly is, a world that seeks to dominate women through masculine violence. The Marquis and Glanville dismiss this truth as a romantic fiction, and Arabella's stalwart belief in this reality becomes a troublesome inconvenience for them.

In the eighteenth century, the shift to silent, solitary reading from reading aloud to others or to oneself obscured the boundary between the world of the literature and the world of the reader, and this shift was believed to cause both moral and physical harm.[18] The censures against private reading of imaginative works, which left readers vulnerable to the dangers of immersion, were not new, but these denunciations were reformulated into the language of medical pathology. "Excessive reading" in the eighteenth century was a threat that reached epidemic proportions. Intemperate reading's danger lay in the combination of physical immobility and the stimulation of the imagination. The Swiss physician Samuel Tissot warned his readers of the "side effects" of this practice, which included inflammation of the stomach and intestines, disorder of the nerves, and fatigue. Men of letters were the most vulnerable to such maladies, leading to the diagnosis of their distinctive disorder, hypochondria.[19] Moreover, solitary reading could potentially corrupt the imagination, resulting in a rejection of empirical reality and a desire for the chimerical. In this way, excessive reading and its concomitant solitary pleasures caused "pallor, anxiety, prostration."[20] Symptoms were exacerbated if the text was a novel and the reader was a woman.[21] Ana Vogrinçic demonstrates the cultural and medical elements to the moral panic centered on early prose fiction: "Broadly, one could divide the reproaches into those ascribing to novels . . . dangerous psychological affects, triggering imitation and inoculating wrong ideas of love and life; and into those referring to the mere habit of novel-reading as a physically harmful waste of time, damaging not only the mind and the morale of readers, but also their eyesight and posture."[22] Charles Povey's *The Virgin in Eden; or, The State of Innocency* (1741) uses the metaphor of poison to describe the harmful effects of titillating novels—in his case, *Pamela*—on the reader's body and spirit: "Had I a Train of Sons and Daughters, and as numerous a Company of Servants as King Solomon, not one of them, by my Consent, should read such Romances of unchaste Love. What tho' some of Pamela's Letters give Hints that may be imitated, does not the Poison contain'd in others destroy all, and give Birth to loose and wandering Imaginations?"[23] What is more, there is no known antidote once this poison has been absorbed. This language, while used metaphorically, is also used literally in medical contexts. The Scottish naval physician Thomas Trotter pronounces full immersion in reading novels as "one of the great causes of nervous affection, even to mental derangement," cautioning that it was "such poison as has no antidote on the shelves of the apothecary."[24] For Povey and Trotter, the use of "poison" to describe the contaminating effect of immersive reading of romances works to describe the pollution of the mind and the body. The transfer of poisonous content from the book to the reader's body can cause irritation to the nerves, with no remedy to neutralize the harmful effects.

In the context of medical ideas on the brain's healthy constitution, the danger of immersive reading limited to the genre of the romance or the novel is compounded when the reader lacks experience that will enable them to exercise sound judgment. For the Swiss physiologist Albrecht von Haller, "the seat of the mind must be where the nerves first begin its formation or origin."[25] Closely aligning with the Galenic theory of the nonnaturals' influence on health, Haller claims that the "integrity or soundness of judgment depends upon a perfect and healthy constitution of the brain," with external factors wielding "considerable influence": "for the air, the way of life, food, and customs, either help or diminish the soundness of judgment, the force of the imagination, and the strength of the memory."[26] To exercise reason, there must be a comparison of two or more ideas, and consideration of the relation of these ideas constitutes judgment: "The principal cause of wisdom and invention lies in a slow examination of the ideas, considered in the relation of all their parts one to another in the mind, while, neglecting all other objects, she is employed with a strong attention only upon that which is under examination." When the mind is restricted, "that efficacy of solitude and darkness" makes a "different calculation," like the "exquisite attention of blind people to the nature of sounds." Error occurs when there is "some neglect in contemplating the whole idea" or "from a less congruous connection" of ideas related by "accident, external causes, or affections."[27] What is more, ideas can be "lodged or engraved not in the mind, but in the body itself, by certain notes or characters, incredible in their minuteness, and infinite in their number, recorded in an inexpressible manner in the medulla of the brain."[28] This description implies that these ideas can reside in the body like a virus, microscopic and multiplying, and parallels the same process of the transmission of toxins in a healthy body described by Povey and Trotter.

In Arabella's case, her notions "from the manner of her life and the objects around her" cultivated a severely myopic worldview. Raised in her father's castle and under his tutelage, she was shrouded in "solitude and darkness" that arrested her social and cognitive development. Understanding this, the Countess becomes Arabella's champion among the catty women in Bath, her support ironically described in chivalric terms: "she resolv'd to rescue her from the ill-natur'd Raillery of her Sex." The Countess defends her when the "Circle of these fair Defamers" throw out "contemptuous Jests" at Arabella, by informing them that "she herself had when very young, been deep read in Romances; and but for an early acquaintance with the world, and being directed to other studies, was likely to have been as much a heroine as Lady Bella" (323). When the Countess attempts to gently persuade Arabella to differentiate the values of romance and the actions that embody them, an approach that Scott Paul Gordon characterizes as "historicizing" the texts, Arabella remained unconvinced, for "romantick Heroism, was deeply rooted in her Heart; it was her habit of thinking, a principle imbib'd from education" (329).[29] In the epistemological "solitude and darkness" of the castle's library, she had assimilated the ideas from her books so thoroughly that both her mind and her emotions, operating in full sympathy with each other, made it very difficult for her to abjure her convictions. By this point in the novel, the poison or the virus of bad reading has done its work, and the Countess's antidote proves ineffective.

## AFFECTIVE EXPERIENCE AND SYMPATHETIC READING

If the brain's healthy development depended on experience and the diverse exposure to ideas, the "Cartesian thought experiment" is dramatized in the inexperienced, sheltered young woman reader as a central concern in *The Female Quixote*.[30] The novel was written and published during the early period of the eighteenth-century phenomenon of sensibility, in which the nerve garnered intense cultural, philosophical, and medical interest. Sympathy—common feeling and harmonious balance—became the structure by which to explain how the mind, body, soul, and society operated.[31] Sympathy also explains how readers can deeply identify and empathize with characters in fiction. Adam Smith's *The Theory of Moral Sentiments* (1759) theorizes that sympathy springs from our inability to directly access how another person feels, so we contribute our own feelings to bridge that gap in our understanding: "By the imagination we place ourselves in his situation, we conceive ourselves enduring all the same torments, we enter as it were into his body, and become in some measure the same person with him, and thence form some idea of his sensations. . . . His agonies, when they are thus brought home to ourselves, when we have thus adopted and made them our own, begin at last to affect us, and we then tremble and shudder at the thought of what he feels."[32] And the same sympathetic process occurs when we read: "Our joy for the deliverance of those heroes of tragedy or romance who interest us, is as sincere as our grief for their distress, and our fellow-feeling with their misery is not more real than that with their happiness."[33] Through sympathy, readers become active participants in the fictional landscape of the narrative, as their feelings correspond with the feelings of characters. For Arabella, her participation in the narratives as a fellow-feeling reader not only has delivered pleasure and escape but has also inculcated a supplementary sense of moral codes for both men and women. In the social world of *The Female Quixote*, where Arabella experiences patriarchal tyranny, female ostracism and ridicule, and male predation, I argue that her high and severe expectations of moral conduct from others (which, as I will demonstrate, are not necessarily unreasonable) protect her from violence and harm.

## VITALISM AND SYMPATHY

But how exactly do our nerves (sites of feeling) and our brains (site of reason) operate in the process of sympathetic reading? For this, I turn to the Edinburgh physiologist Robert Whytt, whose influential theories about the sympathetic body or vitalism provided the medical framework that influenced philosophers of sensibility such as Adam Smith, David Hume, and Francis Hutcheson. According to vitalism, a fluid connection existed between the mind and the body, organs and body parts, and even person to person. Vitalism departed from Cartesian dualism, which posited the separation of soul and body, the idea that inspired the work of mechanists like Herman Boerhaave. As a monistic system, vitalism centered the nerve as the dominant agent responsible for a person's voluntary and involuntary motions.[34] Whytt writes, "There is a remarkable sympathy, by means of the nerves, between the various parts of the body; and now it appears that there is still a more wonderful sympathy between the nervous systems of different persons, whence various motions and morbid symptoms are often transferred, from one to another, without any corporeal contact or infection."[35] In Whytt's view, the nerve redefined what it meant to be human.

I will briefly explain Whytt's premises here as they relate to my reading of Arabella, especially in the ways they determine her reflexive responses to self-preservation. In Whytt's treatise *An Essay on the Vital and Other Involuntary Motions of Animals* (1751), he writes that each nerve corresponded with the whole body and that they "truly act[ed] in a circle," and this entire system was supported by an "immaterial sentient principle," "the source of life, sense and motion, as of reason." This redefinition of the soul governed feeling, motion, and rational faculty and was both unified and immaterial.[36] The sentient principle existed throughout the body, but it principally resided in the brain and nerves: "The soul is not confined to an indivisible point, but must be present at one and the same time, if not in all the parts of the body, yet, at least, wherever the nerves have their origins; i.e., it must be, at least, diffused along a great part of the brain and spinal marrow."[37] The sentient principle's force on the body was inaccessible to the conscious mind, and therefore vital motions were not a direct consequence of our use of reason. Therefore, through the sentient principle, the nervous system operated independently and could regulate itself. In this way, the nervous system's susceptibility and reaction to internal and external stimuli remained unconscious to the person, an early conceptualization of reflex action.[38] In *Physiological Essays* (1761), Whytt continues his argument, insisting that movement is dependent on feeling, using the example of a hiccup interrupted by "sudden fear, joy, or grief."[39] The link between sensibility and the body sets a sympathetic chain throughout, a process brought together by feeling: "Those motions, which are occasioned by stimuli, acting, not on the organs moved, but on distant parts, . . . proceed from that sympathy, which prevails in the nervous system; and must be ascribed to an uneasy sensation in the part irritated, since all consent supposes feeling, and is inexplicable upon any other principle."[40] Whytt expresses undisguised admiration for the body's unification with the mind, feeling, and soul: "But as a system, framed indeed with the greatest art and contrivance; a system! in which the peculiar structure of each part is not more to be admired than the wise and beautiful arrangement of the whole."[41] The significance of Whytt's medical philosophy of organic unity, as Nima Bassiri observes, is the continuity of rational and conscious sensibility: "The boundary between voluntary and involuntary—or mental and vital (or even conscious and unconscious)—had become quite permeable."[42]

The purpose of our "instantaneous motion" in all involuntary motion is "the removal of every thing that irritates, disturbs, or hurts the body."[43] This is why we do not necessarily think about how we can preserve ourselves or our species when we are hungry or thirsty. We feel hunger, so we eat. We feel thirsty, so we drink. There is no conscious intent in these actions. For that reason, the soul "immediately and without any exercise of reason, endeavours by all means and in the most effectual manner, to avoid or get rid of every disagreeable sensation conveyed to it by whatever hurts or annoys the body."[44] Departing from Boerhaave's Cartesianism, Whytt argued that it was the soul, the "immaterial sentient principle," that directed a person's involuntary motion, including actions related to self-preservation. Whytt, who was called the "philosophical doctor," included reflections in his examination of the nerve's workings and the ties between the body and the soul.[45] Most remarkably, his medical observations extended to interpersonal contact, how our own nervous sensibility "reads" and reacts to other people. In his observations on the body's reactions to experiencing or witnessing virtuous or vicious behavior, Whytt seems to be drawing from Hutcheson's philosophy in *Essay on the Nature and Conduct of the Passions and Affections, with Illustrations on the Moral Sense* (1728) on moral sense and sensibility:

> The motions excited by pain or irritation, are so instantaneous, that there can be no time for the exercise of reason, or a comparison of ideas in order to their performance; but they seem to follow as a necessary and immediate consequence of the disagreeable perception. And as the Deity seems to have implanted in our minds a kind of SENSE respecting Morals, whence we approve of some actions, and disapprove of others, almost instantly, and without any previous reasoning about their fitness or unfitness; a faculty of singular use, if not absolutely necessary for securing the interests of virtue among such creatures as men![46]

This idea of human beings endowed with "a kind of sense respecting morals" from God recalls Hutcheson's belief that innate benevolence serves as the universal principle of moral sense, that the public sense's "most natural instinct" is "our Determination to be pleased with the happiness of others, and to be uneasy at their misery."[47] Whytt builds on Hutcheson's philosophy, claiming that motions excited by our moral or public sense happen reflexively and involuntarily.

These explorations into reading practices and the medical-philosophical theories of sympathy during the composition and publication of *The Female Quixote* help provide the framework for how Arabella processed her moral education from privately reading romances and how her affective and intellectual experience from reading such material involuntarily directs her emotional responses in her contact with others. Her body's reaction to vicariously experiencing the violence against women in the novel excited disgust, disapproval, and fear, further shaping the innate moral sense that Whytt and Hutcheson described. If women were imagined to have finer sensibilities and a sharper sensitivity to the nonnaturals based on the physiological difference in their nerves, women's contact with objects (like the romance) that disturb or inflame the passions could threaten their emotional and physical well-being. Arabella's deep immersion in rereading romances imprinted ideas of women's sexual and social vulnerabilities in her mind, and her inexperience and isolation exacerbated her inability to discern reality from fantasy. Furthermore, through sympathetic reading, Arabella became an active participant within the narrative, her feelings corresponding with the feelings of the persecuted women in the novels. Through practice and time, her reading inculcated an intense fear of masculine sexual predation, which trained her nerves in organic unity with the mind and the rest of the body to react reflexively to any imminent threat to herself.

## ROMANCE AS A MODE OF SURVIVAL

With the romance as Arabella's epistemological foundation, she assumes that the world of the novel is an accurate representation of reality, a world that is especially dangerous for women. Male characters, driven by their passions, often act in extremes. Arabella presumes this as a social reality, and this belief dictates her social interactions. In a conversation with her cousin Charlotte, Glanville's sister, Arabella asks if she has had many "adventures," a question to which Charlotte tartly responds in the negative, as she has misunderstood Arabella's use of "adventures" to mean indiscreet sexual relationships. Arabella observes that her cousin is "very happy in this respect, and also very singular," since "there are few young Ladies in the World, who have any Pretensions to Beauty, that have not given Rise to a great many Adventures; and some of them haply fatal." Charlotte points out Arabella's inexperience, emphasizing that young ladies "are not so ready to run away with every man they see." Arabella concurs but takes the argument in a different direction than Charlotte expects: "They do not give their consent to such proceedings; but for all that, they are doubtless run away with many times; for truly there are some men, whose passions are so unbridled, that they will have recourse to the most violent methods to possess themselves of the objects they love. Pray do you remember how often Mandana was run away with?" (88). The princess Mandana whom Arabella references here is from Madeleine de Scudéry's *Artamenes; or, The Grand Cyrus* (1690–1691) and was abducted a staggering eight times, a victim of men's "unbridled" passions.

*Cyrus* has educated Arabella on the way men's passions operate and how women are victimized because of men's inherent inability to control themselves. This belief directly subverts the tenacious medical principles of women's essential frailty in bodily self-regulation. It is men, not women, who cannot help themselves in their experience of passion, necessitating women's self-defense. Women live in a constant state of potential victimhood, and armed with this knowledge, Arabella suspects every man she encounters as a possible abductor or rapist.

While historical evidence suggests that Arabella is less likely to be raped because of her class status, rampant underreporting of rape, perhaps with family reputation as the primary concern to protect rather than the victim, could still place her victimization within the realm of possibility.[48] And to some degree, Arabella's instinct that all men (including her uncle, Sir Charles) carry licentious intent serves as an effective repellant. In one instance, Mr. Tinsel, an arrogant suitor of Arabella who planned to take advantage of her inexperience, insists on barging into her room, causing her to faint. The unexpected and distressing appearance of Tinsel is the disagreeable stimulus that moves Arabella's nerves to react: "seeing Tinsel . . . had got into her chamber, . . . she gave herself over for lost, and fell back in her chair in a swoon" (300). Her reflexive response corresponds with the ways romantic heroines experienced imminent peril, "since all Ladies in the same Circumstances are terrify'd into a fainting Fit, and seldom recover till they are conveniently carried away; and when they awake, find themselves many Miles off in the Power of their Ravisher" (300). Here, the woman's sentient principle reacts reflexively to imminent danger by causing her to lose consciousness. Her nerves reacted in organic unity with her body; the movement of fainting depended on Arabella feeling terror. And, through sympathizing with the women characters in novels, Arabella has developed her nervous mechanisms to be hypervigilant. Arabella obviously misreads the situation, causing confusion for everyone in the household, and yet she is correct in reading Tinsel's capacity for violence when he forced himself past her servant Lucy standing guard by Arabella's room. This hypervigilance proves to be effective; Sir Charles forbids Tinsel from ever visiting the family again, and on the way out, Tinsel exclaims, "since this lady is so apt to think people have a design to ravish her, the wisest thing a man can do is to keep out of her way" (303).

Like Tinsel, many of the men seeking to court Arabella believe they have a unique advantage because of her inexperience. Mr. Hervey, a London gentleman visiting his cousin in the country, is Arabella's first contact with a potential love interest, and their interactions offer the first opportunity for her to apply her romantic learning. Hervey's cousin seeds hope in his mind, suggesting that Arabella's inexperience and solitude would work in his favor (never mind that Arabella's status as the only daughter of a Marquis places her well above his suitability for marriage). Hervey then begins his doomed courtship. Arabella is not insensible of Hervey's attentions, and using the precepts of the romance, she arms herself for his advances.

Riding out with her servants one day, Arabella spots Mr. Hervey approaching, and "her Imagination immediately suggested to her, that this insolent Lover had a Design to seize her Person; and this Thought terrifying her extremely, she gave a loud shriek" (19). Her senses and imagination sympathetically and reflexively activate to protect her against a person she has judged as intending harm. Her moral sense in witnessing what she thinks as impending violence from Hervey is, to use Whytt's words, the "necessary and immediate consequence of the disagreeable perception." She orders her servants to apprehend the mortified man, at which point he asks, "What do you take me for?" Arabella declares, "For a Villain, for a Ravisher, interrupted *Arabella*, who, contrary to all Laws both human and divine, endeavour to possess yourself by Force of a Person whom you are not worthy to serve; and whose Charity and Compassion you have returned with the utmost Ingratitude" (20). Enraged, Hervey demands to be released, threatening to stab her servants in her presence, thus validating her suspicions of his intent for violence. In Wendy Motooka's study of English quixotes that includes Arabella, she observes a phenomenon called "faith of seeing," in which a quixote's belief serves as evidence: "The strength of [Arabella's] belief alone—her unwillingness or inability to see things in any other way—supports her analysis and conclusion."[49] Therefore, through Arabella's myopic lens of judging men to be inclined to sexual violence, Hervey's earlier interest in an affair, then his unexpected appearance, could only be calculated by Arabella's imagination to excite terror. Although she initially gives vent to her terror with a "loud shriek," she recovers herself and "with great Calmness" claims her victory, declaring to Hervey, "you are now wholly in my Power" (20). Thinking of her present and future security, she offers to let him go on the conditions that he never see her again and surrender his weapons for her safety, with which he complies. Sensible of the humiliation once this interaction would be made public ("exposed to the Sneers of his Country Acquaintance"), Hervey departs for London soon thereafter (21). Once again, Arabella's idiosyncratic experience—in reading and social contact—serves to confirm her expectations of male motivation and action and, thus, empowers her to react accordingly.

This early episode with Hervey is fundamental for understanding how Arabella harnesses her sympathetic sensibility and moral education from romances not only to distance herself from predatory men but also to gain temporary authority over them. Though Patricia Meyer Spacks views Arabella as a "victim of desire and fiction," Lennox presents Arabella's delicate female nerves, which Whytt declares to be "more moveable than men," as an empowering system, instead of a debilitating bodily mechanism.[50] Furthermore, her successful application of romantic values and principles only strengthens her worldview.

## HEROIC DISOBEDIENCE: REFUSAL TO BE DISPENSED AS MALE PROPERTY

As I mentioned in the introduction, the path to the comic resolution of marriage and domestic harmony is frequently impeded by women in excess. In *The Female*

*Quixote*, Arabella ironically serves as both the object and the hindrance of the betrothal. Sympathizing with the women characters in the romance, Arabella accepts that marriage is inevitable, "as all the Heroines had done" (27). However, her visceral aversion to the conventionally straightforward arrangement of a husband chosen by her father, what she calls her "heroic disobedience," has been animated by this arrangement's incompatibility with her own romantic vision of securing a loving and faithful husband, only achieved through a prolonged period that tests his merit and virtue. Arabella's insistent refusal and resistance based on the models in the romance is the basis of the Marquis and Glanville's frustrations as well as the humor. She appears to be unreasonable: Glanville does not *seem* particularly despicable, and the Marquis is genuinely affectionate and loving with his only child. But if we recall Barreca's observation that women's humor reclaims certain kinds of control over their own lives and that this humor allows readers perspective on patriarchal culture's absurdities, Arabella's conditions would secure *her* safety in an institution that restricts women's freedoms. Just as her reading has conditioned her nervous responses to men, her potential husband must decondition her fears through time and trials.

Lennox's creation of Arabella as a unique character posited the experiment of an inexperienced young women entering the marriage market whose subjectivity as a victim of potential sexual predation energizes her resistance to gender domination through the conventional courtship rituals of marriage. *The Female Quixote* was published just the year before the Hardwicke Marriage Act of 1754, a law that stipulated certain conditions for a marriage to be legally recognized. Fears of the failure of ecclesiastical courts to curb the growth of clandestine marriages, which threatened the secure transfer of property between families, apparently precipitated the bill's introduction into court. Advocates of this bill argued for its necessity in securing property succession by serving as a deterrent for impulsive young lovers and as a protection against predatory fortune hunters, while opponents claimed that the bill only served the interests of the wealthy by imposing high marriage fees and unnecessary delays. Ruth Perry writes that the act signaled a radical change in public discourse on marriage, that "women's reproductive capacities and sexual conduct had become a matter of public interest and social regulation more than ever before."[51] Lennox was writing at a time when the institution of marriage was becoming increasingly regulated, affecting not only the legal status of what constituted marriage but also the sexual subjectivity of persons looking to marry.

While the Hardwicke Marriage Act ostensibly used the arm of the law to protect women (it did not), Arabella strives to avoid marrying a bad husband through her own volition guided by the moral principles of the romance.[52] Susan Carlile writes, "[Lennox] rewrote the formulaic marriage fantasy with literary women as protagonists who refuse to idealize marriage and cleverly find ways to maneuver independently."[53] Rather than idealizing marriage, Arabella idealizes courtship practices: "She always intended to marry some time or other, as all the Heroines had done, yet she thought such an Event ought to be brought about with an infinite deal of Trouble; and that it was necessary she should pass to this State thro' a great Number of Cares, Disappointments, and Distresses of various Kinds, like them; that her Lover should purchase her with his Sword from a Croud of Rivals; and arrive to the Possession of her Heart by many Years of Services and Fidelity" (27). While the language of property acquisition is used here ("purchase" and "possession"), Arabella's vision of courtship entails her suitor (and herself) undergoing several trials over years as proof that he is worthy of her lifelong partnership and love. Therefore, when the Marquis announced his intention for her marriage to Glanville without this extended campaign for her hand, Arabella's "delicacy was extremely shocked at this abrupt Declaration of her Father [and] could hardly hide her Chagrin" (27). Her "delicacy," recalling the language to describe the fragility and sensitivity of women's nervous constitution, is stimulated by this unwelcome piece of news. Her facial expression naturally manifests the disagreeable sensation of hearing a life-changing mandate from her father. Right after she receives this news, Glanville plants a kiss on Arabella's lips in greeting "with the Freedom of Relation." This kiss "gave her a Disgust that shewed itself immediately in her fair Face, which was overspread with such a Gloom, that the Marquis was quite astonished at it. . . . She not only expressed her Indignation by Frowns, but gave [Glanville] to understand he had mortally offended her" (28). If, for Whytt, movement is dependent on feeling, Arabella's facial responses directly express her displeasure with Glanville's intimate violation on her person. Haller writes, "For the respective muscles, more especially of the voice, face, and eyes, do naturally express the several passions of the mind, so faithfully, that they may even be represented by a painter."[54] In both cases, disagreeable stimuli raise nervous activity in the body, and the face becomes the means by which this displeasure is communicated. Like a painting on a canvas, the face "faithfully" reproduces the internal passions experienced. Arabella's body registers both experiences as a threat to her imagined future and therefore to herself.

While Arabella's reaction genuinely demonstrates her disapproval with the Marquis's decision for her future husband, her sympathetic identification with romantic heroines does not make this turn of events unexpected. She thinks, "What lady in romance ever married the man that was chosen for her? In those cases the remonstrances of a parent are called persecutions; obstinate resistance, constancy and courage; and an aptitude to dislike the person proposed to them, a noble freedom of mind which disdains to love or hate by the caprice of others" (27). Unwavering refusal to this agreement is modeled in the romance as "heroic disobedience" and is Arabella's "noble freedom of mind" in practice. The comic irony of Arabella's "noble freedom of mind" lies in her perspective that she thinks she has the ability to exercise independent judgment, even as we know that "romantick Heroism, was deeply rooted in her Heart" (329), influencing her thoughts, feelings, and actions. And yet, if quixotism functions as a trope to ridicule opposing political values through different political principles, Arabella's application of the high moral codes of the romance allows her a sense of reclaiming autonomy in her own will to love or hate on her own terms and not through the whims of others. Furthermore, the suitability and virtues of the proposed match are not a relevant factor for consideration; the very practice of the Marquis *choosing* a husband for his daughter, removing the daughter's ability to choose for herself, will result in an "aptitude" to immediately despise the potential choice. Arabella's quixotism brings to light the violence of the paternalist model that restricts the freedoms of daughters in their supposed interest. And as the novel develops, the Marquis's own interest in securing his lineage, and the cruelty he exercises to do so, will become clearer to the reader.

Arabella's romantic education ultimately gives her the unique foresight to anticipate male tyranny and violence and the desperate measures she must take to preserve herself. She determines that a coerced marriage arrangement is inevitable, that "all these things must necessarily happen" (35). While she makes it clear that she disapproves of the match with her cousin, who has the temerity to announce his love for her before he has proven this love through years of noble service, Arabella recognizes the futility of relying on his support, that he will ultimately force her into obedience. Furthermore, she believes that Glanville has the power to overcome her, either by indirectly appealing to the Marquis or by direct, brute force: "[The Marquis's] resolution was fixed, and if she did not voluntarily conform to it, she exposed herself to the attempts of a violent and unjust lover, who would either prevail upon the marquis to lay a force upon her inclinations, or make himself master of her person, and never cease persecuting her, till he had obliged her to give him her hand" (34). Glanville had been previously banished by Arabella for the insults she received, which threw her into "an Excess of Anger and Shame" (32). And yet, he continues to appear before her, demonstrating that his desire to satisfy his own needs supersedes respecting hers. Arabella knows that there is no reasoning with men, whose passions govern their bodies and will, and thinks it "both just and reasonable to provide for her own security by a speedy flight" (34). And although there was no literary precedent ("she did not remember to have read of any heroine that voluntarily left her father's house"), she remembers that she is unlike the women who eloped with a "favoured lover," "which would have been highly prejudicial to her glory" (35). She concludes that "there was nothing to hinder her from withdrawing from a tyrannical exertion of parental authority, and the secret machinations of a lover, whose aim was to take away her liberty, either by obliging her to marry him, or by making her a prisoner" (35). Two male agents threaten her freedom, by either a forced marriage or imprisonment, and the only means of survival is escape. And, if she cannot escape one or the other, she can find escape in death. She informs her father that marrying Glanville would be physically violent. She cannot bestow affection on someone she does not love, but she does have the power to kill herself: "Questionless, I know how to die, to avoid the effects of what would be to me the most terrible misfortune in the world" (54).

Arabella absolutely refuses to submit. She will be free, dead or alive. She draws from the resolve of heroines: "I do not yield, either in virtue or courage, to many others of my sex, who, when persecuted like me, have fled to death for relief, I know not why I should be thought less capable of it than they; and if *Artimisa*, *Candace*, and the beautiful daughter of *Cleopatra*, could brave the terrors of death for the sake of the men they loved, there is no question but I also could imitate their courage, to avoid the man I have so much reason to hate" (54). While these women expressed their loyalty with their readiness to die with their imprisoned lovers who had been sentenced to death, Arabella's imitation of them articulates a loyalty to her own self. These heroines found "relief" in death when faced with a life without their lovers; Arabella would find the same release rather than be bound to a life with a man she hated. Even though this self-destructive intent goes against the vitalist view of the immaterial sentient principle's directive for self-preservation, when the state of being itself is harmful, the person can remove themselves from existence.

If the root of Arabella's romantic "honorable disobedience" stems from her inexperience and isolation, exposure to the realities of society should help her disavow her rigid and unrealistic principles. Recall the Countess's remark that her "early acquaintance with the world, and being directed to other studies" expanded her knowledge of social realities. This approach of broadening of experience to develop a healthy brain constitution aligns with Haller's notions that a restricted mind computes logic differently, thus restricting the body to only a singular framework. It is only experience and diversity of study that can cultivate "wisdom and invention." A young person's entrée into society is fundamental for their emotional and intellectual maturity. Still, Glanville wrestles with the advantages of restricting Arabella's movement (and, by extension, her mind) for his own desires.

Arabella's liberty, therefore, remains threatened by Glanville's intentions to claim her as his wife. Arabella wishes Glanville well upon inheriting a third of the Marquis's estate, perhaps imagining that she can finally live out her life as the single woman she desires, a *feme sole*; she had previously expressed to her father that her "first Wish . . . is to live single" (41). Nevertheless, Glanville's passion for Arabella drives him to continue his campaign to win her consent. While he refuses Sir Charles's suggestion to force Arabella to marry Glanville (which shows that the risk of coerced marriage still very much exists as long as a patriarchal head can exert that authority), he privately laments the limitations of the Marquis's control over his daughter: "he would sometimes wish the marquis had laid a stronger injunction upon her in his will to marry him; and regretted the little power his father had over her" (65). His death, "a thousand inconveniences," meant that

Glanville "lost a powerful mediator" (65). Fearing that this window of coercion had closed, Glanville worries that "when she appeared in the World, her Beauty and Fortune would attract a Croud of Admirers, among whom, it was probable, she would find some one more agreeable to her Taste than himself," and "this thought made him extremely uneasy" (65). Glanville would rather not resort to "unjustifiable methods," "to do all that was honorable to obtain her," but his private thoughts reveal that a coerced marriage would be preferable for himself. With her father gone, not only does he have to labor to earn her consent, but he would also be competing with other interested men who, in his mind, might be preferable candidates to Arabella. This insight into Glanville's insecurities upholds Arabella's strong suspicions of men's intent to restrict her freedom. Glanville, above all, preferred for the Marquis to impress Arabella to marry him. Without this "powerful mediator," Glanville's candidacy as her husband is in jeopardy. Recognizing that her freedom of choice increases the chances of finding a more suitable husband for her (perhaps her equal in rank since Glanville is untitled), he becomes more anxious to keep her isolated from the rest of society so he can continue to work on earning her consent without resorting to "unjustifiable methods."

## A QUIXOTIC COURTSHIP

Much of the novel's humor is produced by the discrepancy between the courtship practices of the time and the ostensibly unrealistic way to winning the heroine's heart in the romance. Arabella's basing her moral principles according to the conventions of the romance renders her as an absurd comic figure. Juxtaposed with her cousin Charlotte, Arabella seems parochial and naïve, in need of a broader education to help her disavow her quixotism that makes her so difficult. However, if women's comedy highlights the difference in what they know to be true and what they are *told* to be true, *The Female Quixote* presents conventional courtship practices as ultimately failing to protect women. The father's endorsement only serves himself in the secure transfer of property, and with a short engagement, the potential suitor can feign love and devotion. And knowing that the truth of one's emotions are indelibly marked on the body, a woman on the marriage market will eventually see evidence of a man's sincerity or dissimulation. Stephanie Hershinow describes novices, or inexperienced young women, in the early realist novel as "youthful protagonists" who "in crossing a threshold from private to public life, approach the wider world differently than those understood as already belonging to it," and the misunderstandings of how the novice "reads" a situation "divorces the novice from the society that understands how things 'really' work but, in doing so, grants the novice a position of moral authority from which to understand that society—or even, by comparing it to a more idealistic vision, to improve upon it."[55] The novel's humor is at Arabella's expense, but ironically, her alternate vision, based on the woman's own ability to discern her own and others' emotions, to trust what she *feels* from what she sees, does more to protect her than the preexisting models that serve to secure and satisfy the financial and carnal interests of the men in her life.

Perhaps Glanville expected an easier experience in receiving Arabella's consent for marriage, but it is *he* who misreads Arabella's visual cues that represent her true feelings for him. Although Arabella tells Lucy that Glanville "is no contemptible Person" before their introduction, he makes the mistake of kissing her in greeting. Neither Glanville nor the Marquis is surprised by her response; the former imputes it to her "Country Education," and the latter to "an overscrupulous Modesty" (28). Arabella has shown no inclination in accepting Glanville as her husband, and yet he presumes reciprocation when he announces his love and admiration "with a gentle Pressure of her Hand" (32). His words and unwelcome touch throw "the astonished Arabella into such an Excess of Anger and Shame" that it leaves her speechless (32). Contrary to the "Laws of Gallantry and Respect," in which a lover would suffer "Years in Silence before he declares his Flame to the divine Object that causes it, and then with awful Tremblings, and submissive Prostrations at the Feet of the Offended Fair," Glanville's behavior is a "horrid Violation," provoking a rush of rage within Arabella's body and mind (32). Arabella's reflexive response to highly unwelcome physical contact links sensibility and the body; these nonlinguistic cues of disgust and anger signal how her body interpreted Glanville's touch as a violation. However, Glanville reads Arabella's bodily cues as feigned modesty or as a "Jest," believing that they are both playacting the rituals of courtship. For Arabella, courtship is not a game; her entire self is at stake here, and her visceral responses of repugnance and indignation to Glanville's disregard for her moral principles are authentic.

Arabella's quixotic approach to courtship challenges the accepted practices of her time. She rejects her father's gentle, then forceful, directives to accept Glanville as a suitable husband. A strong example of this is when the Marquis forces her into writing a letter to Glanville to repeal his banishment, though she insists on writing in her own language and expression that makes his coercion clear (40). And because of her inexperience, she does not play the coquette in her contact with men as her cousin Charlotte does. Her strident expectations of virtuous male conduct disarm Glanville and the other men interested in her as their life and educational experiences render them inadequately equipped to meet them. While her romantic notions may seem unreasonable or ridiculous to other characters in the novel, Arabella does not take men's capacity for violence for granted, even including her own father. In a fit of frustrated rage over her disobedience, the Marquis threatens to burn her books (55). Glanville may have fallen "passionately in Love with his charming Cousin" in only a few days, but Arabella remains skeptical, especially after he repeatedly disappoints her (30). *The Female Quixote* underscores the urgency for young women to trust their own judgment and instincts and to erect an emotional defense against suitors on whom their lives and safety may depend.

One way to ensure the integrity of a potential spouse is to prolong courtship and engagement, during which any subterfuge would be discovered, and Arabella's adoption of this approach, based on the heroic examples in the romance, functions as a kind of prophylactic to prevent harm to her health and safety.[56] This delay also serves as a narrative device, as the protraction of Arabella and Glanville's courtship could be due to a sequence of events that Julia Epstein calls "delaying actions," the complications that frustrate the story's ending.[57] The central conflict in most courtship novels is in the entanglement between a young lady's negotiation between her family's demands and her own desires, and as far as we know, the Marquis insists on Glanville's suitability because he is kin. But Arabella's standards for herself are far greater; the lover must prove himself worthy of her hand through noble action, not just because he is endorsed by a male authority figure. After the Marquis commands Glanville to return to the castle, thus nullifying Arabella's banishment, Glanville is determined to win her love by adapting himself to the "Oddity of her Humour": "As he was really passionately in Love with her, he resolved to accommodate himself, as much as possible, to her Taste, and endeavour to gain her Heart by a Behavior most agreeable to her" (46). This change, at first, seems to work in his favor. Arabella notices the alteration in Glanville's conduct "with a great deal of Satisfaction" and begins to speak with him "with the greatest Sweetness and Complaisance," leaning on his arm during their walks together (46). Over time, he has earned the privilege of her conversation and her touch. Though he maintained this friendly distance, Glanville internally experienced turbulent passion: "It was with the greatest Difficulty he restrained himself from telling her a Thousand times a Day that he loved her to Excess" (46). Weeks later, feeling "heartily weary of the Constraint he laid upon himself," he asks her, "What greater signs of Repentance can you desire than this Reformation in my Behavior?" (47). Arabella's answer explicitly makes it clear that declarations of reformation are not enough; there must be clear and visible physiological signs, as well as actions taken by the offender, to demonstrate that the reformation is genuine. Arabella draws from Scudéry's *Artamenes; or, The Grand Cyrus*, which has examples of men who make shallow promises and thus provides Arabella with the benchmarks of false and true reformation:

> Repentance ought to precede reformation. . . . Otherwise there is great room to suspect it is only feigned: and a sincere repentance shows itself in such *visible marks*, that one can hardly be deceived in that which is genuine. I have read of many indiscreet lovers, who not succeeding in their addresses, have pretended to repent, and *acted as you do*; that is, without giving any signs of contrition for the fault they had committed, have eat and slept well, never lost their colour, or grew one bit thinner, by their

> sorrow; but contented themselves with saying they repented; and, without changing their disposition to renew their fault, only concealed their intention, for fear of losing any favourable opportunity of committing it again: but true repentance, as I was saying, not only produces reformation, but the person who is possessed of it *voluntarily punishes himself* for the faults he has been guilty of. Thus Mazares, deeply repenting of the crime his passion for the divine Mandana had forced him to commit; as a punishment, obliged himself to follow the fortune of his glorious rival; obey all his commands; and, fighting under his banners, assist him to gain the possession of his adored mistress. Such a glorious instance of self-denial was, indeed, a sufficient proof of his repentance; and infinitely more convincing than the silence he imposed upon himself with respect to his passion. (47; emphasis added).

In this example, Mazares, one of Mandana's many abductors, is commanded to serve his rival Cyrus as evidence of his penitence. In this model, penance must be undertaken in a voluntary and public expression of pain. Anyone can apologize. Anyone can feign change. For Arabella, penance marks itself on the body, and the test of a man's virtue transpires over years, not weeks. A fraud could not keep up the deceit for that long, and the truth will inevitably reveal itself. In this case, true emotion and true intent mark themselves on the body, visibly seen as genuine expressions.

This approach tests Glanville's character, and he fails spectacularly. He immediately undermines his own progress with Arabella shortly after this speech, proving the efficacy of her courtship philosophy. Arabella earnestly instructs him to read her books to improve himself (thereby fashioning him into a more suitable husband), but instead of reading them, he dissimulates: "He pretended to be deeply engaged in reading, when, in Reality, he was contemplating the surprising Effect these Books had produced in the Mind of his Cousin; who, had she been untainted with the ridiculous Whims they created in her Imagination, was, in his Opinion, one of the most accomplished Ladies in the World" (50). While Glanville is performing the act of reading, he reflects on the contaminating function of the romance, what it had done to Arabella's mind. Arabella, on the other hand, views these books as a gateway to personal improvement. When it becomes clear during a short discussion that Glanville did not do the reading, Arabella realizes that "she had been all this time the Dupe of her Cousin" (51). Glanville's deception is "so glaring a proof of his disrespect" that "she could not find words severe enough to express her resentment" (51–52). Recalling Whytt's ideas on moral sense and sensibility with interpersonal contact, persons "approve of some actions and disapprove of others, almost instantly, and without any previous reasoning about their fitness or unfitness," which is "absolutely necessary for securing the interests of virtue."[58] The incontrovertible evidence of Glanville's patronizing dishonesty instantaneously compels her to banish him from her sight yet again: "she ordered him *instantly* to quit her Chamber" (52; emphasis added). She does not express *how* she feels but expresses the *consequences* of such feelings. In this moment, Arabella learns from "the ridicule to which she had exposed herself" when she opens herself to intimacy (51). Rather than enduring further abuse from "the hated Importunities of a Man she despised" (52), she asserts her power to remove him, leaving him no room for protest or justification. As the novice in *The Female Quixote*, Arabella's inexperienced and isolated status should make her more vulnerable; she knows little of the "real world," after all. However, her continued disappointment with Glanville, even after she allowed him some access of increased intimacy, only confirms what she already knew and felt: Men lie to get what they want.

## PLAYING THE HERO

If the medical establishment's determination of women's physical inability to self-regulate reinforces the patriarchal imperative to police women for their own welfare, *The Female Quixote* forcefully demonstrates that the problem is *not* women's excesses but women's refusal to cooperate through voluntary containment and control. The moral justification for men to make decisions to protect women against others and themselves is questioned when the Marquis and Glanville scheme to manipulate Arabella's feelings toward Glanville to make her more receptive to accepting him as her husband.

There is perhaps no other episode in the novel that so clearly articulates the pernicious capacity of male homosocial desire than the collusion of the Marquis and Glanville in their efforts to present Glanville as a hero. Eve Kosofsky Sedgwick, in her examination of homosociality, defines male desire as the "affective or social force, the glue, even when its manifestation is hostility or hatred or something less emotively charged, that shapes an important relationship."[59] Both the Marquis and Glanville share the same goal regarding Arabella's choice of husband, and they both attribute her books as the obstacle to this goal. Both view the books' damage on Arabella's mind with frustrated rage. Glanville, rather than holding himself accountable for his deceit, "curs[es] *Statira* and *Orontes* a thousand times" and loathes "the Authors of those Books with all the Imprecations his Rage could suggest" (52). And the Marquis, after Arabella's refusal to marry, referencing the bravery of three heroines as her reasoning, threatens to burn her library (55). They both accuse Arabella of being unreasonable, yet they themselves resort to violence if their desires are not met. The misdirected anger toward her books and their authors makes no sense. The impression that these books have made on Arabella's worldview is permanent (even with her "reformation" at the novel's end, which I explore later). Destroying the books will not magically undo the way Arabella thinks of herself and of men. The intent to burn her books, then, become symbolic in how it represents male dominance and imminent male violence. Glanville, however, would rather not turn to "unjustifiable methods" to win her consent. And yet he absolutely exploits the violent potential of the tyrannical father for his own benefit.

The two men's collusion to present Glanville more favorably to Arabella, their dupe, makes clearer the triangular structure of the three. Arabella is what Lévi Strauss calls the "conduit of a relationship," in which she is the object of the exchange between men in marriage.[60] As the Marquis's only child and daughter, Arabella acts as a channel for the secure transmission of wealth within the family. As far as we know, the only reason the Marquis insists on Glanville's suitability to be Arabella's husband is his kinship tie as her cousin. The maintenance of wealth in the patriarchal hegemonic economy relies on male homosocial bonds, as Heidi Hartmann explains: "Patriarchy [is] a set of social relations between men, which have a material base, and which, though hierarchical, establish or create interdependence and solidarity among men that enable them to dominate women."[61] The Marquis considers himself at the apex of this familial hierarchy, and it is through his authority that he commands the transfer of erotic emotions that would facilitate a conjugal union. He proclaims as much to Arabella: "[Glanville's] presumption [to declare his intentions] . . . was authorised by me: therefore, know, Bella, that I not only *permit* him to love you, but I also expect you should endeavour to return his affection; and look upon him as the man whom I design for your husband" (39; emphasis added). Their previous nonsexual father-daughter relationship takes an incestuous bent when she reaches marriageable status. An endogamous marriage, along with the reproductive sexual acts between cousins associated with it, ensures the security of the bloodline, with the husband/nephew standing as the embodiment and extension of the father/uncle. In this way, though Arabella is the property of the Marquis to "give away," to use Lynda Boose's words, he would not lose her (and, by extension, himself and his wealth) in an endogamous arrangement.[62]

Both the Marquis and Glanville derive a perverse pleasure from manipulating Arabella's emotions. The Marquis, "resolved to cure Arabella of her whims," transfers his enjoyment of burning the books onto Glanville: "I have seized upon some of them, pursued he, smiling; and you may, if you please, wreak your spite upon these authors of your disgrace, by burning them yourself" (56). The Marquis, perhaps in half jest, attributes Arabella's loss of respect for Glanville to these authors, responsible for shaping her exacting standards of masculine virtue, standards Glanville fails to meet. The Marquis mildly assigns blame on his nephew for drawing himself into "a terrible Dilemma," but he primarily holds the books and their authors responsible. Glanville quips back, "Though I have all the reason in the world to be enraged with that incendiary Statira . . . for the mischief she has done me; yet I cannot consent to put such an affront upon my cousin, as to burn her favourite books: and now I think of it, my lord . . . I'll endeavour to make a merit with Lady Bella by saving them; therefore spare them, at my request, and let me carry them to her. I shall be quite unhappy till we are friends again" (56). Glanville doubles down on his deceptive behavior, seeing an opportunity to project himself in a more favorable light to Arabella by playing the hero to the father's cruelty.

And Glanville certainly performs the hero, not only by saving her beloved books from the flames but also by assuming a matching expression. Finding her in a "Deluge of Tears," he privately judges the cause of her weeping to be "ridiculous" (56). Glanville patronizes Arabella, treating her with apparent kindness, but betrays an air of intellectual and gendered superiority. He believes himself to know how the real world works and sees his cousin as tragically deluded. What is more, for Whytt, a person's "most natural instinct" is to "be pleased with the happiness of others, and to be uneasy at their misery"; Glanville's callous response to Arabella's tears reveals a break in his own moral sense, further demonstrating his inability to act as a virtuous partner for her. Instead of sympathizing with another's distress, as Arabella does consistently throughout the novel, Glanville contemptuously dismisses her feelings with ridicule. Still, these tears have made some impact on Glanville, and "assuming . . . a countenance as sad as he was able," he returns the books to her, claiming that "it was with much difficulty he prevailed upon the Marquis not to burn them immediately" (57). The ruse works; Arabella's expression "brightened into a smile of pleasing surprise at the sight of her recovered treasure" (57). She repeals his banishment for "this little service," though this act does not "cancel [his] past offences" (57). Glanville confirms the success of his ruse with the Marquis: "nothing could have happened more fortunate for him, than his intended disposal of his daughter's books, since it had proved the means of restoring him to her favor" (57). "Fortunate for him" underscores the benefit Glanville receives from the Marquis's threat of violence toward his own daughter and, more importantly, shows the reader Arabella's correct judgment of his duplicitous character.

The scheme is effective, but only to a certain degree. Arabella allows Glanville back into her company, but she still maintains a skeptical and guarded mien. Again, the lover she will eventually accept as her husband will need to prove his worth through years of devotion and loyalty. The "little service" of rescuing the books is not enough for that yet. Her smile of "pleasing surprise" quickly turns into "significant frowns" that "gave Glanville to understand his stay was displeasing" (57). Her smile may briefly betray her emotional interiority, but Arabella recovers herself to preserve physical and emotional distance from Glanville through bodily expression. She has learned from his first offense of lying to be wary of allowing any man to become too intimate with her. Later, when Glanville questions Arabella's suspicions of his ill designs, she says, "It is not strange if I cannot consent to acquit you in my Apprehensions, till I have more certain Confirmation of your Innocence, than your bare Testimony only; which, at present, has not all the

Weight with me it had some time ago" (114). His "bare Testimony" is insufficient to prove his innocence; "certain Confirmation" is necessary to trust him, especially after catching him in a lie.

This extensive analysis of the Marquis and Glanville's homosocial collusion could be read simply as a humorous episode in the novel. Arabella, as the dupe, falls for the scheme laid out between her father and cousin (albeit with some reservations). Glanville becomes the "good guy" standing against the Marquis's cruelty. However, reading this episode through the lens of the comic subversion of women's humor, I argue that the joke lands squarely on the absurdity of men, the lengths they will go for control and their sadistic glee in executing these schemes. The threat to destroy her dead mother's books imply a latent, or even imminent, violence as a consequence of disobedience. And as the novel progresses, this violence becomes a more appealing means to "cure" Arabella in her "madness," which manifests in her persistent refusal to yield what little power she has over herself.

## MADNESS AS PUBLIC; OR, THE LIMITS OF MASCULINE IMAGINATION (AGAIN)

The problem of Arabella's quixotism takes on a more pressing and public dimension when the Marquis dies, and Sir Charles, her uncle and Glanville's father, has been appointed as her guardian. At first, Glanville worried over his competition when Arabella enters the social scene, that she would find someone "more agreeable to her Taste than himself" (65). Now, his concern centers on his and his family's reputation if she were to remain as herself. Arabella's venturing out into the open world should have developed her brain through the exposure of new ideas that could supplant the outdated (and troublesome) notions brought on by her romantic learning. And yet Arabella holds fast to her principles, which embarrasses the entire family, especially Glanville, whom Sir Charles holds responsible for controlling Arabella. On the difficulty of disengaging powerfully lodged ideas in persons, Haller writes, "The strength and duration of an idea depends upon its being either unusual, of a strong action, or greatly conducing either to increase or lessen our felicity; or, lastly from being joined with great attention from the mind, and often repeated; all of which circumstances being conjoined, may render the species so strong to the mind, that she will afterwards receive the perception of them, as if they came from external objects, in the manner we observe in mad people."[63] Arabella's case may well have been a complete example drawn from Haller's book: The "unusual" and "strong action" of the romance taught Arabella the path to "felicity," free from harm, ideas often "repeated" from rereading. Her successful application of these principles, "circumstances being conjoined," reaffirms the truth of these novels' reality. This "species" of ideas lodges itself so strongly and inflexibly in the minds of mad persons. Any challenge to the order of things—especially intimations that men not only fail to protect women but also actively seek to harm them—causes an uneasy disruption to the domestic harmony that depends on women's silence and compliance. While *The Female Quixote* demonstrates the empowering expressions of the romance for women, the novel's progress toward its conclusion shows that this liberating existence outside the realities of the "real world" is unsustainable.

After a public incident in which two men thought Arabella's brain "disturbed," Glanville realizes with more clarity that he is conflicted over her fantastical flaws and her virtues and the consequences of greater public exposure for his reputation. Arabella's "romantic notions" are not substantial enough to "lessen a Passion which every Sight of her so much the more confirmed," yet "*his* Happiness depended upon curing her of her romantic Notions" (117; emphasis added). Glanville may not be wrong in his assessment of a favorable solution: If Arabella were "cured," she would let go of the delusions she operated under and would accept him as her husband, thereby circumventing the years and years of loyal devotion she previously required from him. It is worth noting that Arabella's happiness is not a consideration here, underscoring the selfishness of Glanville's intentions. And abandoning her is out of the question, as "he feared it was impossible to help loving her" (117). His passion prevents him from disentangling himself from her. He struggles with whether increased social contact will lead to a cure or further embarrassment: "Sometimes he fancied company, and an acquaintance with the world, would produce the alteration he wished: yet he dreaded to see her exposed to ridicule by her fantastical behaviour, and become the jest of persons who were not possessed of half her understanding" (117). While it seems that Glanville is concerned for Arabella's well-being here as the possible target of gossip, he seems more interested in the consequences for his reputation if or when they marry. Arabella could gain a reputation for being an unusual woman at best or a mad one at worst, and either mark on her image could negatively impact his own. Her willfulness is the killjoy of his happiness. The killjoy brings unhappiness to herself by refusing to grant the happiness of others. And so, if Arabella refuses to relinquish control, a problem that she brings to herself, this problem must be solved by force for her own good and the good of everyone else.

The men in the novel tend to intuitively diagnose Arabella's "madness" when they struggle to comprehend her behavior or speech. Sir Charles simply assumes that her disobliging manner could only be attributed to mental disease: "he was so lost in Wonder and Confusion at a Behavior for which he was not able to assign any other Cause than Madness" (200). He tells his son, "She behaved in a very impertinent Manner to me, . . . complained of my harsh Treatment of her; and said several other Things, which, because of her uncommon Style, I could not perfectly understand; yet they seemed shocking; and upon the Whole, treated me so rudely, that I am determined to leave her to herself, and trouble my Head no more about her" (201). Sir Charles operates emotively, deducing from Arabella's mode and style of speech rather than the substance that her words *seem* "shocking." His complete incomprehension, however, gives him leave to conclude, "It is not fit she should have the Management of herself" (201). His anger, frustration, and helplessness in his interactions with his niece provoke a consequential judgment that she is incapable of self-autonomy. His impatience with her incomprehensibility reaches its apex when he learns of Arabella's behavior in full view of the public at the pleasure gardens and "concludes she was absolutely mad, and held a short debate with himself, Whether he ought not to bring a Commission of Lunacy against her, rather than marry her to his Son, whom he was persuaded could never be happy with a Wife so unaccountably absurd" (339). Glanville, thrown into agonies at this suggestion, feels the pressure from his father, who asks him to consider "the absurdity of her behaviour, and the ridicule to which she exposed herself wherever she went, . . . whether in a wife he could think those follies supportable, which in a mistress occasioned him so much confusion" (339). Sir Charles is thinking about the future in store for Glanville, whether he can endure his wife's "follies" under constant public ridicule.

Sir Charles's threat to confine Arabella, most likely in a private madhouse, would not be unusual. Andrew Scull writes in his study of the origins and establishment of Victorian asylums in England that in the eighteenth century, only a small fraction of people diagnosed as insane were incarcerated, the most violent patients and members of propertied classes whose "mental peculiarities threatened their relations with social or financial ruin."[64] Indeed, there was a high demand by people belonging to Sir Charles's station for a system of private care that would relieve them from the burden of mad relations and to sequester these relations from public view.[65] Sir Charles was not alone in considering isolating Arabella as recourse to prevent family embarrassment. His daughter Charlotte tartly offers her pity that "Protestant nunneries" did not exist, for "her Cousin ought to be confin'd in one of those places, and never suffer'd to see any company, by which means she would avoid exposing herself" (314). While readers of the novel witness the embarrassment the family endures due to Arabella's singularity, her behavior stemming from delirium does not seem to warrant serious medical treatment for insanity.[66] Michael McDonald identifies "extravagance, incoherence, incomprehensibility, menace, and ungovernable rage" as characteristics that fit the prevailing stereotypes of madness in the period.[67] Arabella's extravagance of speech, in the "high flown style" of romance, can be incomprehensible for some, yet the Countess and Glanville's rival Sir George, both having read romances, can understand her and can even speak the same language in return. Still, her "mental peculiarities" on public display are enough to justify tucking her away out of everyone's sight, if only to continue the cycle of female victimization brought on by masculine anxiety. Her overt inscrutability in speech and conduct distresses the males in the narrative who seek to possess—and, correspondingly, to know—her body.

Though Sir Charles is prepared to deliver Arabella to a madhouse, Glanville desperately hopes for a cure, albeit with some hesitation. Leland E. Warren notes Glanville's earlier ambivalence regarding "curing her of her romantic Notions." Glanville initially wishes to delay Arabella's "awakening," for it may make her less of the woman he loves, that "the brilliance he perceives in Arabella is in part a function of her separation from a reality that might repress desire."[68] In other words, in rousing from her fever dream of the romance, she might realize that she does not want him. Though he plays along as the pining lover at the castle, he soon grows desperate for Arabella to be silent in the public spaces of Bath and London. Sir Charles warns his son of the onerous responsibility of protecting the family's reputation: "It was his business to produce a reformation in her; for, added he, notwithstanding the immense fortune she will bring you, I should be sorry to have a Daughter-in-law, for whom I should blush as often as she opens her mouth" (64). Even the "immense fortune" amassed from their union would not be enough to protect the family from public shame. Upon marriage, Arabella's status as a *feme covert* would entail the surrender of her linguistic autonomy as well as her wealth. It would become her husband's "business" to direct her speech and manner into the acceptable modes determined by the patriarchal institutions of that society that seek to maintain gender domination.

It would then become Glanville's responsibility to reeducate, or uneducate, Arabella of the learning she acquired from her father's library. She is often viewed as incomplete or imperfect, and her cure would make her whole, make her perfect. Sir Charles tells Glanville, "When you are her husband, you may probably find the means of curing her of those little follies, which at present are conspicuous enough; but, being occasioned by a country education, and a perfect ignorance of the world, the instruction, which then you will not scruple to give her, and which, from a husband, without any offence to her delicacy, she may receive, may reform her conduct; and make her behavior as complete, as, it must be confessed, both her person and mind now are" (180). As noted earlier, Arabella's behavior would not have fit the eighteenth-century stereotype of a madwoman. But, as Scull explains, there was a major shift in the principal paradigm of insanity, away from highlighting its "demonological, non-human, animalistic" features (seen in Bertha Mason's madness and propensity for violence in Charlotte Bronte's *Jane Eyre* [1847], for example) toward a naturalistic viewpoint that considered the madman as presenting a "defective human mechanism" that was possibly treatable.[69] This "defective human mechanism" is believed to produce the "little follies" in Arabella's brain. Once that defect is corrected, all will be well. "To be absolutely perfect," Glanville exclaims, "I must cure her of that singularity" (197). And recalling

Deutsch and Nussbaum, women's bodily difference is compared with deformity, "so that women are, by their very nature, deemed to be defective." Defect is used as a category to reinforce the normative engine of systems of domination. Arabella's "singularity," her only defect, must be cured so Glanville can dominate her body. The plot's trajectory is shaped by the ultimate resolution of satisfying male desire for compliance and silence embodied by the heroine's body and mind. Conformation to enact a heteronormative narrative that is no story at all, like the Countess's, acts as a palliative to the male frustration caused by the inaccessibility of women's mind, bodies, and knowledge. Unaccountable behavior cannot be understood, only silenced or modified to acceptable ways of knowing and comprehension. And if that does not work, difficult women can always be sent far away to restore the domestic order.

## ARABELLA'S REFORMATION AS PENANCE

In the end, Glanville does facilitate a cure for Arabella's "singularity" through an intermediary.[70] We are presented with the learned divine in whom Glanville rests his hopes for Arabella's "reformation" after she, like Clelia, attempts to swim across a river to escape imagined rapists and nearly drowns. She confides in the Doctor about her motives for these "rash and vain-glorious" actions: "the Danger she was in of being carry'd away, the Parity of her Circumstances then with *Clelia*, and her emulous Desire of doing as much to preserve her Honour as that renown'd *Roman* Lady did for hers" (366–367). Confounded by her speech, the Doctor listens to Glanville's explanation of "the disorders romances had occasioned in her imagination," to which the Doctor promises to "spare no endeavours to rescue [her noble mind] from so shocking a delusion" (367). The method to cure Arabella's mind takes on a surgical precision: The illness is located in her disordered brain and must be cut out to save her life.

The clergyman, confident in his intellectual authority, feels both admiration and anxiety for Arabella, but he later determines that her mind possesses the strong constitution to bear the weight of his arguments. The ensuing dialogue covers different questions about the appropriate role of narrative as a didactic tool and source of knowledge of the world. The novel's conclusion with Arabella's reformation has often been read as proof of masculine reason triumphing over feminine fantasy (a problematic binary that has been properly interrogated), but I read the persuasiveness of the Doctor's rhetoric as not from his strength of logic but from its pathos. Arabella declares, "My heart yields to the force of Truth" (381). But which (or whose) "truth" is she referring to?

Arabella challenges the Doctor to prove that these histories are "fictions," "absurd," and "criminal" (374). He meets this challenge by arguing that these stories that purportedly took place two thousand years ago only emerged in the last century and only from French authors who drew haphazardly from history (375, 378). He proclaims that these romances are absurd not only because they are unrealistic but also because they set up misleading expectations for readers in the real world, especially for the young and inexperienced (378–379). Finally, these romances are "criminal" since they teach the wrong kind of passion that is fundamentally fueled by revenge and love:

> These books soften the heart to love, and harden it to murder. That they teach women to exact vengeance, and men to execute it; teach women to expect not only worship, but the dreadful worship of human sacrifices. Every page of these volumes is filled with such extravagance of praise, and expressions of obedience, as one human being ought not to hear from another; or with accounts of battles, in which thousands are slaughtered for no other purpose than to gain a smile from the haughty beauty, who sits a calm spectatress of the ruin and desolation, bloodshed and misery, incited by herself. (381)

In the Doctor's assessment, the violence in the world of the romance is provoked by the sadistic pleasure of women in authority. Remarkably, a man telling a young woman (or any woman) that rape and abduction are nonsensical fictions is ridiculous.

It is presumably this final point that moves Arabella to reflect with guilt and shame, realizing that her past actions could have endangered others: "I now wonder how the blaze of enthusiastic bravery could hinder me from remarking, with abhorrence, the crime of deliberate unnecessary bloodshed . . . and fear that I have already made some approaches to the crime of encouraging violence and revenge" (381). In the same way that Lady Booby's and Lady Bellaston's passions find counterbalance, Arabella's feelings of guilt and shame operate as a way of control. She attributes her choices to her own desire for legacy, to avoid historical oblivion: "I tremble indeed to think how nearly I have approached the brink of murder, when I thought myself only consulting my own glory" (381). Indeed, an illustrious life has directed her acting and thinking, as she had previously criticized the fashionable ladies of Bath and London who spent their time in "trifling Amusements" and had interrogated the meaninglessness of such a life: "How mean and contemptible a Figure must a Life spent in such idle Amusements make in History? Or rather, Are not such Persons always buried in Oblivion, and can any Pen be found who would condescend to record such inconsiderable Actions?" (279). A brief exposure to the realities of women in high society was enough to show the moral superiority of the romance heroines she emulates. Warren writes, "She can be someone in a nonexistent world or she can become like the females she sees around her and be a nobody in the real world."[71] Arabella had struggled to avoid the fate that she saw exemplified in the Countess, who, as Catherine A. Craft observes, "personifies that doom to which Arabella must succumb."[72] When the Countess is asked by her ingénue to relate her "Adventures," she narrates the cookie-cutter, predictable heteronormative narrative of "Women of the same Rank, who have a moderate Share of Sense, Prudence and Virtue" (327). That is to say, the Countess cannot relate any adventures under the rigid standards of a patriarchal society that places moral responsibilities on women. The traditional story of the virtuous woman is not a story at all, especially compared to the exciting lives of the female heroines in romances, for the virtuous woman's body does not belong to herself.

And in fairness, Arabella mischaracterizes herself here. She might adopt an imperious mien and regularly deploys the sentence of banishment to men who have offended her rules of conduct, but she has hardly "approached the brink of murder." In fact, she has rescinded these sentences or commanded Glanville and Hervey to live when she believed they were at risk of death from heartbreak, demonstrating clemency. Even though she has claimed that "the Blood that is shed for a Lady enhances the Value of her charms" (128) and has ordered Glanville to murder Edward if he does not confess and absolve her cousin of conspiring with him, no blood has been spilled on her account.

In fact, the only person in the novel who has been moved by love and revenge to physically harm another is Glanville. Toward the novel's end, he discovers that Sir George has orchestrated a complicated plot to villainize Glanville in Arabella's eyes. "Fir'd almost to Madness" and "vowing Revenge upon Sir George, execrating Romance, and cursing his own Stupidity," he hatches a plan to catch Sir George in the act of seducing his cousin (354). Soon after, Glanville "came running like a Madman" to Sir George and Charlotte (whom he mistakes for Arabella) and, "actuated by an irresistible Fury," runs Sir George through with his sword (357). When Arabella misreads a situation, there is no real physical harm done. When Glanville does the same, a man is skewered. The Doctor holds the "haughty beauty" responsible for the loss of lives in the landscape of the novel, but in the world inside and outside *The Female Quixote*, it is the excess of men's passions and their inability to appropriately regulate these passions that inflict real and consequential violence. Arabella's impulsive or deliberate choices in any present moment come from removing anything or anyone that could do harm to herself or other women, while Glanville's motivation here is to reclaim the shame from a rival, a selfish act born from a bruised ego.

Having called Arabella's mental rehabilitation a "Miracle" performed by the good Doctor, Glanville "fancied to himself the most ravishing Delight from conversing with his lovely Cousin, now recovered to the free Use of all her noble Powers of Reason" (382). The complex irony here rests on Glanville imagining the "ravishing Delight" in speaking with a woman who has "recovered" the "free Use" of reason. He is enraptured with the future of easy conversations with Arabella, now that her "silly follies" have been excised from her imagination. She is no longer difficult, a killjoy. As I mentioned earlier, Arabella's tenacious fear of rape, of

"Ravishers," played a major part in her obstinate refusal to let go of the ideas implanted in her brain. Now, her "free Use" of reason indicates a symbolic surrender to the masculine penetration of her mind. Social intercourse through language is ultimately also sexual intercourse, once Arabella yields to Glanville's suit of marriage: "To give you myself . . . with all my remaining Imperfections, is making you but a poor Present in return for the Obligations your generous Affection has laid me under to you" (383). The fever dream of romance has been broken. The "cure" brought about by male authority is to ignore her body's own signals. In the end, the novel consigns Arabella to Glanville's hands instead of a madhouse, and all her adventures, imagined or real, come to a close in servitude and penance to a husband, a tragic ending of domestic imprisonment that she has so heroically resisted.

# CODA

## Surgical Violence as a Tool of Masculine Dominance in *Poor Things* (2023)

THROUGHOUT *BODY LANGUAGE*, I HAVE explored how the eighteenth-century comic novel uses the pathologized female body in its ambivalent deployment of humor. On the conservative end, women's excess becomes an object of ridicule when the leaky woman presumes agency beyond her social reality. Shamela and Winifred Jenkins affect a literary sensibility that transcends their servant class. Ladies Booby and Bellaston attempt to assert sexual agency like male libertines. Mrs. Shandy and Mrs. Trunnion presume to know their own pregnant bodies better than their husbands and male obstetricians do. Arabella is confident that she understands the world through her romantic learning. Ironically, these women need *reform* to preserve the patriarchal tradition. On the radical end, these novels critique how medicine fails to explain how women's bodies work, and how marriage, almost always prescribed as a cure for women's excesses, falls short for women. The humor in these narratives reveals a palpable anxiety of the shortcomings of prevailing patriarchal systems in absolute domination and for the possibilities of gender liberation, a counternarrative of women's embodiment, agency, and selfhood defined outside or without the institutionalized efforts of medicine and marriage. One can envision how these novels, to use a scientific term, experimented with new ways of thinking and doing things, to imagine an alternate present and future.

In closing, I move forward and backward with the film *Poor Things* (2023), considering these same themes by examining the problem of women's sexuality through the medical lens and in the comic mode. *Poor Things*, a genre-defying film with science fiction, gothic, and comic elements set in Victorian-ish Europe, features Bella Baxter, an adult woman whose brain has been transplanted from her own fetus by the scientist and physician Godwin Baxter ("God") after she has thrown herself from a bridge. The film's main thought experiment is the portrayal of a woman reborn with a subjectivity free from the social pressures that prohibit gender agency. She gets to start all over again in an adult woman's body with the memories of her old life scraped clean. All the instruction on how to be a proper woman, to be virtuous, chaste, and restrained, and the consequences of failing to meet these standards, is gone. And aligning with the comic tradition, sex is central in the film. Bella discovers the joys of masturbation in her early development and engages in unbridled sexual pleasure (what she charmingly calls "furious jumping") with her rakish lover Wedderburn, strangers, and brothel clients. Freed from the bondage of gendered conditioning, Bella openly pursues sexual pleasure. Sex is not separated from her intellectual and emotional development; in fact, sex becomes a kind of epistemology for Bella, who learns about herself and her social reality (although the film brings up troubling questions of consent since Bella's "mental age and her body are not quite synchronized," as Baxter puts it). She discovers that women's sexuality is only a problem for certain kinds of men, men like her previous life's husband, General Alfred (Alfie) Blessington, whose "life is dedicated to the taking of territory."[1] To fix the problem, husbands like Alfie turn to the extreme "cure" of surgical violence.

*Body Language* has explored how the representation of women's bodies through physical, psychological, and emotional embodiment is rooted in sexed and reproductive difference and how this difference became the justification for masculine domination in all areas of life in the eighteenth century. By the end of the century, scientific and medical discourse shaped a cruder and more inflexible biological essentialism that prescribed specific social roles for women (domesticity and motherhood) based on their physical (possessing a uterus and ovaries) and mental (fragile) attributes. By the 1800s, physicians not only accepted this difference as *fact* but also grew convinced of the direct, sympathetic connection between a woman's brain and her uterus.[2] The circumstantial and inferential research of Marshall Hall, Thomas Laycock, and Johannes Müller on the sympathetic nervous system confirmed women's increased vulnerability to emotional disorder and mental illness originating from the turbulence of the female reproductive system.[3] Each stage of a woman's life brought new threats to her well-being. Andrew Scull and Diane Favreau explain, "Puberty, pregnancy, parturition, lactation, menstruation, and the menopause, each added to the constant shock and strain on the bodily system, prompting, in all too many cases, the wreck of the intellect, the collapse of the will, and the dissolution of all semblance of self-control."[4] The idea that the uterus was the root of mental and physical disease meant that the therapeutic intervention for female insanity was administered by both neurologists *and* gynecologists. And with the development of anesthesia in the 1840s and the acceptance of antisepsis in the 1860s, routine use of invasive surgery became the norm in obstetrical and gynecological treatments.[5] In the eighteenth century, women who were suspected of suffering from an incurable mental illness were committed to asylums; in Lennox's *The Female Quixote*, Sir Charles had threatened this measure to Glanville if he failed to cure Arabella's apparent insanity. By the time when *Poor Things* is set, surgical violence in the forms of hysterectomy (removal of all or some parts of the uterus) and clitoridectomy (excision of the clitoris) was practiced by both psychiatrists and gynecologists to remedy mental and emotional disease.

It is unsurprising, then, that Alfie turns to surgical violence to force Bella to submit. The doctor asks Alfie, "Do you want just clitoral hood, or glans as well?" Alfie answers, "The whole infernal packet." The doctor assures him, "It will calm her no end" (92–93). A wife's resistance and refusal to her husband is perceived as nervous hysteria. Rather than acknowledging the oppressive conditions that marriage imposes on women, as Anne Finch and Lady Wortley Montagu had insisted, doctors and husbands interpreted the wife's intractability as a symptom of mental disorder caused by disturbances from her reproductive system, including the genitals. While ancient medical theories of hysteria, from Hippocrates to Galen, attributed the source of illness to the womb, external pudenda became included as part of the "whole infernal packet" in the nineteenth century.

Women's sexuality became an object of increasing scrutiny in the nineteenth century, and any aberrant behavior could be remedied with medical or surgical intervention. Female-specific disorders, including nymphomania, masturbation, "moral insanity," hysteria, "menstrual madness," and the ill-defined neurasthenia, were considered life-threatening, justifying the excision of parts from women's reproductive systems.[6] The French neurologist Jean-Martin Charcot, who specialized in hysteria and hypnotism, believed that most mental illnesses in women developed from abnormalities of the female external genitalia.[7] Clitoridectomy was promoted as the most effective treatment by the highly influential physician and Royal College of Surgeons fellow Isaac Baker Brown of London and the French neurologist Charles Brown-Séquard in Paris. In 1866, Brown published *On the Curability of Certain Forms of Insanity, Epilepsy, Catalepsy and Hysteria in Females*, which advocated for clitoridectomy as a cure for all the disorders outlined earlier, as well as for painful and heavy periods, depression, dementia, and even death.[8] Aligning with the principle of reflex irritability, Charles Brown-Séquard claimed that injuries to the nervous system might stem from overexcitement of the peripheral nerves.[9] Baker Brown traced the connection between his patients' nervous illness and the practice of masturbation, referring to it as the "peripheral excitement of the pudic nerve." While medical texts on the dangers of onanism and the threat of masturbatory insanity had long been circulating by the early nineteenth century, Baker Brown found the existing (and excruciatingly painful) remedy of cauterizing the clitoris to be superficial and temporary to "destroy such deep-seated nerve irritation."[10] To recall Alfie's words, "the whole infernal packet" must be removed.

While Baker Brown applauded his own "success" in curing women of nervous irritation through clitoridectomies, closer scrutiny of the historical context presents a more sinister view. In Baker Brown's collection of cases, several female patients looked to take advantage of the new Matrimonial Causes Act of 1857, which reformed divorce law. Prior to this law, divorce proceedings could only go through the ecclesiastical courts. The new act made secular divorce a possibility (though it still did not treat men's and women's grounds for divorce equally).[11] Consequently, women who pursued legal separation from their husbands were diagnosed with "incipient mania." These women's decisions to live a single life were construed as a symptom of a developing mental illness characterized by overexcitement and excess. In Case 48, for example, Mrs. S.M. grew "a great distaste for her husband . . . and [for] cohabitation with him. [Baker Brown] pursued the usual surgical treatment, which was followed by uninterrupted success; and after two months' treatment, she returned to her husband, resumed cohabitation, and stated that all her distaste had disappeared; soon became pregnant, resumed her place at the head of her table, and became a happy and healthy wife and mother." He concluded that marital harmony could be reestablished through this course, precluding "a judicial separation of husband and wife, with all the attendant domestic miseries."[12] It is noteworthy that the proof of the treatment's effectiveness is expressed in terms of the patient's identity in relation to her husband and in her capacity to give birth and raise his children. The cure was deemed successful *because* she embraced her roles as "incipient mania," which had manifested in her previous rejection of them.

*Poor Things* makes the narrow patriarchal definition of domestic harmony visible through the violence of the husband. Bella is curious to know of her previous life as Alfie's wife, Victoria, and elects to return to the Blessington estate, where she quickly discovers his cruelty. Alfie condemns her past behavior and aggrandizes his own compassion: "Marriage is a constant challenge; some we bend to, some we bend to us. I will try to forgive you for the whoring, your sexual hysteria was often out of hand, and also for the killing of our unborn child. In fact, when I list how you've wronged me Jesus Christ himself would probably beat your head in with a bat. You are blessed with a forgiving husband" (91). He declares that her full recovery will necessitate household imprisonment and that if she tries to leave, he "will have to shoot [her] in the back of the fucking head." Bella confirms, "So I am a prisoner?" Alfie replies, "This conversation has gone down an unfortunate route. I am sure you will be as happy as you were before." "As I was before? When I threw myself from a bridge?" (92). The dark humor in that last line lies in the obvious incongruity between Alfie's belief that Victoria was actually happy and the reality that she had tried to end her life while they were married. For Alfie, the sexual hysteria was the problem, not the uninhabitable conditions of marriage. His misogynistic myopia cannot conceive of a reality outside of himself. He is not the problem. She, in her possession of a messy, leaky body, is the problem that is breaking up the home. As a "forgiving husband," he understands that women, as delicate and fragile creatures at the mercy of their disordered bodily systems, require a moral male guardian to ensure their safety and well-being. Having been disembodied as Victoria (literally), Bella sees the truth behind the repressive regime of marriage without the learned sentimentality of a wife's love and duty. "Growing" without the years and years of patriarchal indoctrination that readies girls for unquestioned subjugation in domestic life, Bella can call out the bullshit. To repeat Regina Barreca's view, "Humor allows us to gain perspective by ridiculing the implicit insanities of patriarchal culture."[13] The comic disparity between what Bella knows to be true and what she is told to be the truth by Alfie underscores the tenuous substantiation for masculine domination.

And in seeing the truth for herself, Bella refuses to continue her domestic duties as Victoria Blessington, which Alfie and the doctor view as a manifestation of her sexual hysteria, warranting surgical intervention. When she insists on leaving, "having now ascertained why [she] threw [herself] from a bridge," after overhearing his conversation with the doctor, Alfie delivers this lecture: "The root of the problem is between your legs and I will have it off and it will not distract and divert you anymore. A man spends his life wrangling his sexual compulsions, it's a curse, and yet in some ways his life's work. A woman's life's work is children, I intend to rid you of that infernal packet between your legs and plant a seed straight after" (94). Alfie's speech could very well be a dramatization of Mr. S.M. of Case 48. Alfie reinforces the belief system that men are naturally hypersexual beings who must learn to control their urges and that women's sexuality should only be for reproductive purpose to secure the future of the patrilineal line. If Bella refuses to accept her "life's work," she will be forced to endure the surgical removal of the site of pleasure and be forced to give birth. Londa Schiebinger's study on how gender structures knowledge and power in medicine and science explains how, by the end of the eighteenth century, European anatomists started to represent sex bodies with specific life objectives: "physical and intellectual strength for a man, motherhood for the woman."[14] The influence of scientific and medical discourse licensed and *naturalized* gender identification according to physical and mental attributes, precisely in the ways Alfie lays out their roles as husband and wife. By disobeying her husband's commands, by bluntly explaining that men or marriage is the problem, by trying to leave marriage through death, Bella/Victoria can only be diagnosed as hysterical. The seat of this illness lay in her reproductive system, and correction required excision.

What is more, Bella's sexual history with Wedderburn and with brothel clients might be construed by nineteenth-century physicians as the behavior of a nymphomaniac, what Alfie calls "her whoring" and "sexual hysteria." In the nineteenth century, nymphomania was described as desiring or having too much sex or too much masturbation and often overlapped with hysteria diagnoses.[15] "Too much" usually meant a woman's indulging in sexual desire that exceeds that of her husband's and enjoying sexual pleasure by herself (and, in some cases, with other women). Yet again, masculine anxiety—the emasculation of the husband's dominance through his sexual prowess—drives the engines of the patriarchal systems of marriage and medicine. In medical case studies, nymphomania reinforced the concept of unmanageable female sexuality for the women patients and for their caretakers. The concept of nymphomania also violated the normative biological facts that viewed women as modest sexual beings. Even minor transgressions of what constituted acceptable feminine modesty, like flirting, wearing perfume, or wearing jewelry, could be (and were) classified as pathological.[16] Gynecologists held onto the belief that nymphomania was marked on the body by hypertrophy of the clitoris, even though a study published in 1840 refuted this idea.[17] Baker Brown celebrated the permanent results of clitoridectomy as treatment: "in no case am I so certain of a permanent cure, . . . for I have never after my treatment seen a recurrence of the disease."[18] Genital excision was forwarded as a panacea for diseases causing women to be difficult wives, to permanently inhibit sexual desires considered immodest or immoral.

In Bella's brief time in the Blessington home, masculine violence is wielded as a threat to female bodily autonomy, first as imprisonment, then surgical violence, and finally with a pistol. Notwithstanding Alfie's threat, Bella delegitimizes his power through her unbothered affect and speech: "I will keep my new life and my lovely old clitoris thank you. So if you'd call for a carriage for me." Drawing his gun, Alfie replies, "They talk and talk, and at some point there is nothing left but to pull a gun. It is the way with women" (94). Alfie's choice to point his pistol at Bella is framed as a last resort, that *she* cannot be reasoned with. This frustration is similar to the Marquis's threat of force in *The Female Quixote* if Arabella does not quietly submit to his demand that she marry her cousin, but instead of books as the cause of her intractability, the source of Alfie's problems is between Bella's legs. His condescending remark that "it is the way with women" is Alfie speaking of women, indirectly to Bella, and of men's duties to discipline their wives. Not only does Alfie normalize men's recourse to violence as something that has to be done, but he also shifts the blame on the wife herself. He would not have had to pull his gun if she just stopped talking and did what he knows is good for her. What is good for her is ultimately only what is good for him. If husbands draw their power from the false dichotomy of gender based on essentialist biology, then a wife's refusal to acknowledge the warrant of such power opens alternative possibilities, undermining the entire structure that girds gender disparity and dispossession. Bella's calm pronouncement that she will keep *her* life and *her* "lovely old clitoris" exercises her right to bodily agency. Although Alfie tells her that his life is "dedicated to the taking of territory," Bella drily retorts, "I am not territory" (94). If men's identity depends on their ability to perform the gendered expectations of domination and aggression, their wives' resistance renders them impotent.

And in a rather heavy-handed ironic turn, Alfie shoots himself in the foot after Bella throws the chloroform-laced martini in his face. Dying from exsanguination, Alfie is taken by Bella to Baxter's lab to try to save his life. Her fiancé and God's assistant, Max McCandles, pauses and remarks, "Bella, if he lives . . . I sense he is not a man who will stop." Bella replies, "I will not watch him bleed to death Max, but I agree, he could do with improvement" (95). In the final act, medicine, the weapon intended to be used by the husband as a means of surgical control, becomes the means to resolve the problem of the husband without murder, improving him by replacing his brain, the seat of his aggression, with the docile brain of a goat.

True to the comic tradition, the film concludes with domestic harmony. Bella forgives the dying Baxter for withholding the truth of her creation. Characters deserving of happiness gather in the garden: Bella, McCandles, the retired sex worker Toinette, the housekeeper Prim, and the new "experiment" Felicity. Bella inherits Baxter's wealth, allowing her to freely pursue a career in medicine. The material futures of these characters are secured, including Alfie's, who is seen on all fours bleating and eating grass.

Alfie's grotesque surgical transformation is laughable because it diminishes him to nothing. He thinks himself superior, as a husband, lord, and military man, dominant in the domestic, the political, and the imperialist spheres. Wielding violence through the pistol and his proximity to the surgeon, he imagines himself with infinite power to maintain his dominance. Immanuel Kant defines laughter as "an affection arising from a strained expectation being suddenly reduced to nothing," a reappraisal of the comic's incongruity theory.[19] Kant understands laughter as a sudden revelation of our own unimportance. Kant's theory contrasts with Thomas Hobbes's more popular contention that laughter arises from a "sudden glory arising from some sudden conception of some eminency in ourselves; by comparison with the infirmity of others, or with our own formerly."[20] For Hobbes, laughter is inherently aggressive; we experience a sudden and pleasant feeling of superiority. The film, I believe, takes a Kantian approach to laughter, critiquing the Hobbesian perspective. Alfie's undisguised triumph with his humiliating prank on a maidservant is not funny, at least not for us today. Additionally, Bella's compassion for the suffering of others, albeit enacted naïvely, demonstrates the film's moral center. Kant's view serves as a kind of social polemic against the ruling class, whose dominance and ascendency are not consequences of natural or biological privilege but of a sustained, systematic, aptly resourced violent campaign. Alfie's comeuppance into a man-goat is funny because, in the end, his status ultimately means nothing.

In the film's comic representations of a woman in excess and anxious masculinity, *Poor Things* thematically aligns with the novels discussed in this book. Women's difference—from their blood to their nerves to their genitals—continues to be the apologia for denying women bodily and reproductive autonomy. Just two years before the film's release, the United States Supreme Court overturned *Roe v. Wade*, effectively nullifying the constitutional right to abortion. In the following year, conservative Christian lawyers affiliated with the Alliance Defending Freedom (ADF), the same group that wrote the model for the overturning of *Roe v. Wade*, requested a Texas federal judge for a nationwide ban on mifepristone, a pill used in half of the abortions in the country. Although the U.S. Court of Appeals for the Fifth Circuit upheld the Food and Drug Administration's 2000 approval of the pill, the Supreme Court heard arguments in the case—*FDA v. Alliance for Hippocratic Medicine*—in March 2024 and issued their unanimous decision to dismiss the case on the basis that the plaintiffs did not have legal standing to bring this challenge to the Court.[21] Notably, the plaintiffs in this case were doctors who were opposed to abortion by the right to freedom of conscience; although these doctors *are not required to prescribe mifepristone*, they argued that they have standing, or the legal right, to sue.[22] As a conservative Christian legal advocacy group, the ADF claims to defend the sanctity of heterosexual marital union and the institution of the family in all its litigious efforts. In this current political moment, we bear witness, yet again, to efforts from the medical establishment to adjudicate ostensible gender difference under the dominant ideology of the family. For now, the federal courts have protected women's access to safe abortion medication, but it is likely that this case could come back on the docket with different plaintiffs with legal standing.[23] The unresolved tensions between women's bodily autonomy and their place in the family—dramatized in the eighteenth-century comic novel and in contemporary films like *Poor Things*—underscore the ongoing question of women's freedom to choose.

# ACKNOWLEDGMENTS

This book—and, in many ways, my interest in eighteenth-century studies—would not have been possible without Kathy Lubey. She introduced me to Fielding and Sterne in my very first term at St. John's University, and never did I imagine that I would laugh so hard in class. Her infectious enthusiasm in and outside the classroom had a profound and lasting impact on my own interest in the early novel and sexuality and gender studies. Her encouragement as professor, dissertation advisor, mentor, and friend has sustained me throughout the years; I will always treasure our conversations and laughter over meals and martinis throughout New York City. Kathy's commitment to good cooking and good writing can be encapsulated in the time she lugged the very heavy *New York Times Cookbook* as my graduation gift on the subway and streets of Manhattan. I aspire to be the spirited writer, teacher, and colleague that she has been for me and for our community. I would also like to thank my dissertation readers, Granville Ganter, Steve Mentz, and Melissa Mowry, whose expertise and thoughtful reviews helped refine the stickier bits on servant literacy that was the foundation of chapter 1.

I count myself very lucky to have landed a tenure-track post at Queensborough Community College (CUNY) right after graduate school. The PSC-CUNY research award gave me the time and resources to continue working on this book. Additional funding from The Book Completion Award, the William P. Kelly Fellowship Award, and the Faculty Fellowship Publication Program (FFPP)—all through CUNY—granted me additional support to design and execute this writing project as untenured faculty. I am especially grateful to my FFPP group leader, Anahi Viladrich, and my fellow participants for helping me think through and, most importantly, finish the book proposal that was the first step in making this project real. Four QCC English Department chairs—Linda Reesman, David Humphries, Jennifer Maloy, and Margot Edlin—have been stalwart advocates of my research goals throughout the years. The friendship of my English Department colleagues, especially Leah Anderst, Aliza Atik, Robin Ford, George Fragopoulos, Susan Jacobowitz, Cara Murray, William Ryan (a fellow *dix-huitièmiste*), Mark Schiebe, Kerri-Ann Smith, Irvin Weathersby, and John Yi, has helped me see this project through, from writing reviews to listening to me complain about the process. I am always grateful for the patient support of the English Department administrative support staff and the librarians at the Kurt R. Schmeller Library.

I am thankful for the unrelenting efforts of our union, the Professional Staff Congress, for its continued support of faculty research and for campaigning for more equitable conditions at CUNY. And I thank my students at QCC who have laughed at my mom jokes, ironically or not, and have cheered me on throughout this journey.

I have found comfort and community as a member of the American Society of Eighteenth-Century Studies (ASECS). Even at my most insecure, imposture-syndrome-ridden self, Kathy Lubey encouraged me to submit my earliest panel proposal for an ASECS conference in graduate school, and I thank her for the gentle, but persistent, push to join this community. I have presented portions of this book at several ASECS and its regional conferences, where fellow panelists and audience members have helped me refine my project's argument. Rebecca Shapiro invited me to join "The Doctor Is In" mentoring program, where I forged a friendship with Danielle Spratt and Adela Ramos. I appreciate Eugenia Zuroski and Kimberly Takahata's faith in me to cochair the Race and Empire Caucus with the fantastic Rebekah Mitsein. The inimitable Tita Chico introduced me to the team at *The Eighteenth Century: Theory and Interpretation*, giving me my first opportunity to edit a collection with many of the important voices in our community. Stephanie Hershinow, then chair of the Columbia University Seminar on Eighteenth-Century European Culture, graciously offered the time and space for me to present my muddiest chapter to a group of kindhearted intellectuals whose insightful input has been instrumental in its final shape. My *Transits* big brother, Jason Farr, has warmly shared his generosity and expertise; from presenting as a guest speaker for my QCC students (prepandemic!) to crafting the ASECS signature Gemini cocktail to reading this manuscript, Jason has been a model of support and compassion. I thank Kirsten Saxton for inviting me into the incredible circle of funny women in the Write With Aphra Writing Group. My first meeting with Bethany Qualls at the ASECS convention in Denver could very well be the first scene of a meet-cute in a biddie comedy. Emily Friedman, Kate Ozment, Megan Peiser, Carrie Shanafelt, and the rest of the Space Cats have staunchly supported my writing and my ranting. Many thanks to the medical humanities folks, especially Travis Chi Wing Lau, Matthew Reznicek, and Miriam Wallace, whose work has helped me think more carefully about my own. Before the great academic exodus of Academic Twitter, many IRL and online colleagues have kept me going in spiritual and online solidarity.

I am deeply indebted to the team at Bucknell University Press, especially Mona Narain and Miriam Wallace, who invited me to submit my book for the *Transits* series. Suzanne Guiod and Pam Dailey have been so kind and accommodating in helping me navigate the unfamiliar and terrifying arena of monograph publication. The anonymous readers of my manuscript provided thoughtful, encouraging, and attentive reports that have helped me shape this book to be much better than I thought it could be.

In the Philippines, I was raised in a culture that valued community and collaboration, and I am so thankful for my neighbors, friends, and kin who have supported me and my family while I wrote this book. The Tamayo and Alves clans, both of which have greatly expanded since I started this enterprise, have given me love, purpose, and fully booked weekend schedules away from work.

This book project is as old as my younger child, and I am deeply indebted to the people in my life who have cared for my children so I could write: My parents, Polly and Joseph Tamayo; my in-laws, Ana Maria and Luciano Alves; my late and beloved Lola, Añumada Catarman; my sister, Kirsten Tamayo; my sister-in-law, Fatima Alves; and the staff at the YMCA Early Learning Center have all lovingly looked after my children so this working parent could write. The circle of mothers in my life who picked up my kids when I was running late from campus, took turns carpooling for sports practices, and arranged playdates and parties will always be in my heart.

Tiffany Malloy, my ride-or-die, has accompanied me through the joys and disappointments of undergraduate and graduate school. She has saved my life in so many ways, and I am forever grateful to the universe algorithm that landed us in the same freshman French class. Our friendship has endured long past the headache we both got on that first day trying to follow French for two hours.

My parents have been a major influence on my work ethic and ambitions. Although I did not ultimately end up in medicine, my physician father's collection of medical textbooks piqued my very early interest in the field. Between shifts at the hospital and the clinic, he helped me learn to read medical terminology I was absolutely not equipped to comprehend as a preschooler. My mother, who earned her way into a medical profession against unthinkable odds, showed me that a woman's identity could encompass both career and family. Both, and our ancestors before them, continue to inspire me as a professor and as a parent.

Daily walks with Comet and Jackson provided both a break and the time for creative incubation whenever I was stuck with writing. Both dogs have been a solid part of my writing community; napping nearby while I write, they have never left me alone during this project. And from what I hear, their impromptu cameos during Zoom meetings have earned them a celebrity status with students and faculty.

My children, Jonathan and James, just like the novelists examined in this book, remind me every day to never take things too seriously, that there is humor in anything and everything. They have amassed an admirably expansive comic-strip collection in their libraries; it has been a joy to see them appreciate wit, wisecracks, and comedy in any form and even more so when they share them with me.

Without them, perhaps this book would have been finished much sooner, but my life would have been less full.

As much as I have doubted myself writing this book, Dave never lost faith in my ability to push it through to publication. He cheers every win, sympathizes with every loss, and has loved me every step of the way since high school. To his credit, he knew I would end up professoring in English way before I did. Without his material and emotional support, it would have taken me much longer to finish graduate school and even longer to finish this book. He is, and will always be, the love of my life. I hope I make Dave and my children proud, and this book is lovingly dedicated to the three of them.

A section of chapter 1 appeared as "'What Pleasure We Scullers Have': Humor, Menstruation, and Literacy in Smollett's *Humphry Clinker*," in *Journal for Eighteenth-Century Studies* 38, no. 3 (2015): 349–360. The first half of chapter 2 was published as "'Whither Doth This Violent Passion Hurry Us?': Hysterical Language and Desiring Women in Henry Fielding's *Joseph Andrews*," in *Eighteenth-Century Fiction* 32, no. 4 (2020): 559–578. Both articles are reprinted with permission.

The author expresses appreciation to the Schoff Fund at the University Seminars, Columbia University, for their help in this publication. Material in this work was presented to the University Seminar on Eighteenth-Century European Culture.

# NOTES

## INTRODUCTION

1. Henry Fielding, *"Joseph Andrews" and "Shamela,"* ed. Martin C. Battestin (Boston: Houghton Mifflin, 1961), 262. Subsequent references are to this edition and are cited parenthetically in the text.
2. As the number of domestic servants who were able to read grew steadily in eighteenth-century Britain, writers became aware of how the text can affect moral character. There is evidence that a range of men and women servants read for pleasure and self-improvement. Jan Fergus, "Provincial Servants' Reading in the Late Eighteenth Century," in *The Practice and Representation of Reading in England*, ed. Helen Small and Naomi Tadmor (Cambridge: Cambridge University Press, 1996), 202–225.
3. Jean Astruc, *A Treatise on All the Diseases Incident to Women Containing an Account of Their Causes, Differences, Symptoms, Diagnostics, Prognostics and Cure, Translated from a Manuscript of the Author's Lectures Read at Paris, 1740* (London: M. Cooper, 1743), 59. Although French, Astruc enjoyed widespread popularity among both English and Scottish professors and practitioners of midwifery. His works and theories were cited in lectures given by Thomas Denman, Alexander Hamilton, William Osborne, William Smellie, and Thomas Young.
4. "Science," as used in the modern sense, gained its current meaning in the nineteenth century. Here, I am using the word anachronistically, in reference to the range of research, experimentation, and activity in natural philosophy.
5. Karen Harvey's examination of how laypeople understood physical, affective, mental and spiritual embodiment offers a counternarrative from the gendered view of medical discourse. See Karen Harvey, "Epochs of Embodiment: Men, Women and the Material Body," *Journal for Eighteenth-Century Studies* 42, no. 4 (2019): 455–469.
6. The most recent examination of "race-medicine" in the context of eighteenth-century British empire is Suman Seth's *Difference and Disease: Medicine, Race, and the Eighteenth-Century British Empire* (Cambridge: Cambridge University Press, 2020).
7. See Susan S. Lanser, "Novel (Lesbian) Subjects: The Sexual History of Form," *Novel: A Forum on Fiction* 42 (2009): 497–503; and Lanser, "Sapphic Dialogics: Historical Narratology and the Sexuality of Form," in *Postclassical Narratology: New Essays*, ed. Monika Fludernik and Jan Alber (Columbus: Ohio State University Press, 2010), 186–205.
8. Lauren Berlant and Michael Warner, "Sex in Public," *Critical Inquiry* 24 (1998): 548, 552.
9. While queer scholarship remains a minoritized subfield in eighteenth-century studies, there is a rich production of research that recuperates queer histories and practices, moving the discipline in more intersectional positionings. On queerness and disability, see Katherine B. Crawford, *Eunuchs and Castrati: Disability and Normativity in Early Modern Europe* (London: Routledge, 2018); Jason Farr, *Novel Bodies: Disability and Sexuality in Eighteenth-Century British Literature* (Lewisburg, PA: Bucknell University Press, 2019); Travis Chi Wing Lau, "Defoe before Immunity: A Prophylactic *Journal of the Plague Year*," *Digital Defoe* 11 (2019): 23–39; Chris Mounsey, *Sight Correction: Vision and Blindness in Eighteenth-Century Britain* (Charlottesville: University of Virginia Press, 2019); Jarred Wiehe, "No Penis? No Problem: Intersections of Queerness and Disability in Laurence

Sterne's *The Life and Opinions of Tristram Shandy, Gentleman*," *The Eighteenth Century* 58, no. 2 (2017): 177–193. On transgender studies, see Julia Ftacek, "Jonathan Swift and the Transgender Classroom," *Journal for Eighteenth-Century Studies* 43, no. 3 (2020): 303–314; Anson Koch-Rein, "*Trans*-lating the Monster: Transgender Affect and *Frankenstein*," *LIT: Literature Interpretation Theory* 30, no. 1 (2019): 44–61; Jane Manion, *Female Husbands: A Trans History* (Cambridge: Cambridge University Press, 2020); Geoffrey Sill, "Robinson's Transgender Voyage: or, Burlesquing Crusoe," *Robinson Crusoe after 300 Years*, ed. Andreas K. E. Mueller and Glynis Ridley (Lewisburg, PA: Bucknell University Press, 2021), 27–60; Jolene Zigarovich, "Transing the Gothic," *in TransGothic in Literature and Culture* (London: Routledge, 2017), 1–22. On race and queerness, see Jeremy Chow, "Mare Mortis: Blackness, Ecology, & 'Kinlessness' in Neville's *The Isle of Pines*," *Atlantic Studies* 18, no. 2 (2021): 1–17; and Kara Keeling, *Queer Times, Black Futures* (New York: New York University Press, 2019).

10. Thomas Laqueur, "Orgasm, Generation, and the Politics of Reproductive Biology," in *The Making of the Modern Body: Sexuality and Society in the Nineteenth Century*, ed. Catherine Gallagher and Thomas Laqueur (Berkeley: University of California Press, 1987), 18.
11. Felicity Nussbaum, *Torrid Zones: Maternity, Sexuality, and Empire in Eighteenth-Century English Narratives* (Baltimore: Johns Hopkins University Press, 1995), 23.
12. Quoted in Laqueur, "Orgasms," 18.
13. Ludmilla Jordanova, *Sexual Visions: Images of Gender in Science and Medicine between the Eighteenth and Twentieth Centuries* (Madison: University of Wisconsin Press, 1989), 24.
14. John Bender, *Ends of Enlightenment* (Stanford, CA: Stanford University Press, 2012), 40.
15. Mary Lindemann, *Medicine and Society in Early Modern Europe* (New York: Cambridge University Press, 2010), 110–112.
16. Biology and Gender Study Group, "The Importance of Feminist Critique for Contemporary Cell Biology," in *Feminism and Science*, ed. Nancy Tuana (Bloomington: Indiana University Press, 1989), 172–187.
17. Lynda Birke, *Women, Feminism, and Biology: The Feminist Challenge* (New York: Methuen, 1986), 114–117.
18. See Christina Larner, *Enemies of God: The Witch-Hunt in Scotland* (Baltimore: Johns Hopkins University Press, 1981).
19. Jordanova, *Sexual Visions*, 24–25.
20. Evelyn Fox Keller, *Reflections on Gender and Science* (New Haven, CT: Yale University Press, 1985), 3.
21. Londa Schiebinger, *The Mind Has No Sex? Women in the Origins of Modern Science* (Cambridge, MA: Harvard University Press, 1989), 191.
22. Pierre Roussel, *Système physique et moral de la femme, ou Tableau philosophique de la constitution, de l'état organique, du temperament, des moeurs, et des fonctions propres au sexe* (Paris, 1775), 2.
23. Jacob Ackermann, *Über den Einfluss des Geschlechts-Unterschiedes auf Ausbildung und Heilung von Krankheiten* (Stendal, 1829), 28–30.
24. Schiebinger, *Mind Has No Sex?*, 191.
25. In the past few decades, women's studies has led to radical responses of received truths in the histories of science, medicine, and literature. Feminist scholars and their work—like Ludmilla Jordanova's *Sexual Visions* (1989) and Lynda Birke's *Women, Feminism, and Biology* (1986)—have disputed the traditional notions of reason and normality, authorship and authority, sex relations, and sensibility. These critics have contended that these categories must be viewed as constructions, not as natural and immutable, the products of masculinist ideologies. Schiebinger's *The Mind Has No Sex?* examines the transformations of the female and the identification of modern femininity and sexuality.
26. Lesley Dean-Jones, *Women's Bodies in Classical Greek Science* (Oxford, UK: Clarendon, 1996), 107.

27. Laura Gowing, *Common Bodies: Women, Touch, and Power in Seventeenth-Century England* (New Haven, CT: Yale University Press, 2003), 79.
28. Lynda Birke, *Feminism and the Biological Body* (New Brunswick, NJ: Rutgers University Press, 2000), 176.
29. On the link between illnesses and individual identity, see Roy Porter and Dorothy Porter, *In Sickness and in Health: The British Experience 1650–1850* (London: Fourth Estate, 1988).
30. See Andrew Wear, *Knowledge and Practice in English Medicine 1550–1680* (Cambridge: Cambridge University Press, 2000), 154–209.
31. On the broad range of medical theories and treatments, see Lester S. King, *The Medical World of the Eighteenth Century* (Chicago: University of Chicago Press, 1958), 1–58; and Wear, *Knowledge and Practice*, 78–82. On the connections between mind, morals, and body, see Porter and Porter, *In Sickness and in Health*, 60–75; Wear, *Knowledge and Practice*, 178–184, 281–288.
32. See Porter and Porter, *In Sickness and in Health*, 21–42; Wear, *Knowledge and Practice*, 178–184.
33. Peter Lewis Allen, *The Wages of Sin: Sex and Disease, Past and Present* (Chicago: University of Chicago Press, 2000); Marie E. McAllister, "'Only to Sink Deeper': Venereal Disease in *Sense and Sensibility*," *Eighteenth-Century Fiction* 17, no. 1 (2004): 87–101; Linda Merians, ed., *The Secret Malady: Venereal Disease in Eighteenth-Century Britain and France* (Lexington: University Press of Kentucky, 1996); Gail Kern Paster, *The Body Embarrassed: Drama and the Disciplines of Shame in Early Modern England* (Ithaca, NY: Cornell University Press, 1993); Claude Quétel, *History of Syphilis*, trans., Judith Braddock and Brian Pike (Cambridge, UK: Polity, 1990); Kevin Siena, "'The Venereal Disease,' 1500–1800," in *The Routledge History of Sex and the Body, 1500 to the Present*, ed. Sarah Toulalan and Kate Fisher (London: Routledge, 2013), 463–478; Michael Stolberg, "Self-Pollution, Moral Reform, and the Venereal Trade: Notes on the Sources and Historical Context of *Onania* (1716)," *Journal of the History of Sexuality* 9, no. 1 (2000): 37–61.
34. Though distinctly different genres, I am placing "comedy" and "satire" in the same generic category in their means of using laughter to criticize human foibles and vices.
35. Thomas D'Urfey, *Scandalum magnatum, or, Potapski's Case, A Satyr against Polish Oppression* (London, 1682), 8.
36. John Dryden, *An Evening's Love or the Mockastrologer*, in *The Works of John Dryden*, vol. 10, ed. Maximillian G. Novak and George R. Guffey (Berkeley: University of California Press, 1970), 203.
37. John Dryden, *A Discourse Concerning the Original and Progress of Satire*, in *The Satires of Decimus Junius Juvenalis: Translated into English Verse by Mr. Dryden and Several Other Eminent Hands* (London: Jacob Tonson, 1693), 32.
38. Magda Romanska and Alan Ackerman, introduction to *Reader in Comedy: An Anthology of Theory and Criticism*, ed. Magda Romanska and Alan Ackerman (London: Bloomsbury, 2017), 12.
39. Romanska and Ackerman, introduction to *Reader in Comedy*, 12.
40. Mikhail Bakhtin, *Rabelais and His World*, trans. Hélène Iswolsky (Bloomington: Indiana University Press, 1984), 26.
41. Elizabeth Grosz, *Volatile Bodies: Toward a Corporeal Feminism* (Bloomington: Indiana University Press, 1994), 203.
42. Birke, *Women, Feminism, and Biology*, 160.
43. Birke, *Women, Feminism, and Biology*, 109.
44. Nancy Tuana, *The Less Noble Sex: Scientific, Religious and Philosophical Conceptions of Woman's Nature* (Bloomington: Indiana University Press, 1993), 22.
45. Essaka Joshua, "Disability and Deformity: Function Impairment and Aesthetics in the Long Eighteenth Century," in *The Cambridge Companion to Literature and Disability*, ed. Clare Barker and Stuart Murray (Cambridge: Cambridge University Press, 2018), 47.

46. Helen Deutsch and Felicity Nussbaum, introduction to *"Defects": Engendering the Modern Body*, ed. Helen Deutsch and Felicity Nussbaum (Ann Arbor: University of Michigan Press, 2000), 11.
47. *Beauty's Triumph, or, the Superiority of the Fair Sex Invariably Proved* (London, J. Robinson, 1751), 151.
48. Quoted in Romanska and Ackerman, introduction to *Reader in Comedy*, 12.
49. James Beattie, "Essay on Laughter and Ludicrous Composition," in *Essays*, 3rd ed. (London: Edward and Charles Dilly, 1779), 321–486; Frances Hutcheson, *Reflections upon Laughter, and Remarks on the Fable of the Bees* (Glasgow: R. Urie, 1750); Immanuel Kant, *Critique of Judgement*, trans. James Creed Meredith and Nicholas Walker (Oxford: Oxford University Press, 2007).
50. Simon Dickie, *Cruelty and Laughter: Forgotten Comic Literature and the Unsentimental Eighteenth Century* (Chicago: University of Chicago Press, 2014), 190–249, 220–221.
51. Laurence Sterne, *The Life and Opinions of Tristram Shandy* (1759), ed. Ian Campbell Ross (Oxford: Oxford University Press, 2000), 539. Subsequent references are to this edition and are cited parenthetically in the text.
52. Romanska and Ackerman, introduction to *Reader in Comedy*, 6.
53. Lisa Hopkins, "Marriage as Comic Closure," in *The Shakespearean Marriage* (London: Palgrave Macmillan, 1998), 16–33.
54. Northrop Frye, *Anatomy of Criticism, Four Essays* (Princeton, NJ: Princeton University Press, 1957).
55. Kant, *Critique of Judgment*; William Hazlitt, "Lecture I—Introductory: On Wit and Humour," in *Lectures on the Comic Writers, Etc. of Great Britain*, ed A. R. Waller and Arnold Glover (London: J. M. Dent, 1903); Ted Cohen, *Jokes: Philosophical Thoughts on Joking Matters* (Chicago: University of Chicago Press, 1999); Sigmund Freud, *Jokes and Their Relation to the Unconscious* (London: Penguin, 2002); John Limon, *Stand-Up Comedy in Theory, or, Abjection in America* (Durham, NC: Duke University Press, 2000).
56. Lauren Berlant and Sianne Ngai, "Comedy Has Issues," *Critical Inquiry* 43, no. 2 (2017): 239.
57. Berlant and Ngai, "Comedy Has Issues," 233.
58. Grosz, *Volatile Bodies*, 19.
59. Paster, *Body Embarrassed*, 64–112 (chapter 2, "Laudable Blood: Bleeding, Difference, and Humoral Embarrassment").
60. Bryan Turner, *The Body and Society: Explorations in Social Theory* (Thousand Oaks, CA: Sage, 1996), 1.

## CHAPTER 1 — LEAKY WRITINGS AND LEAKY BODIES IN HENRY FIELDING'S *SHAMELA* (1741) AND TOBIAS SMOLLETT'S *HUMPHRY CLINKER* (1771)

1. John Freind, *Emmenologia*, trans. Thomas Dale (London: T. Cox, 1729), 132–135.
2. Bakhtin, *Rabelais and His World*, 26.
3. B. Turner, *Body and Society*, 1.
4. Jared S. Richman, "The Other King's Speech: Elocution and the Politics of Disability in Georgian Britain," *The Eighteenth Century* 59, no. 3 (2018): 279–304.
5. Most recently, Heather Meek's work on the multiple understandings and representations of blood in the eighteenth century demonstrates the ways in which women's recorded experiences with medical interventions and bloodletting challenge the incorrigible leakiness of women's bodies. Heather Meek, "'Meanders of [the] Purple Flood': Blood and Bloodletting in Eighteenth-Century Literature and Medicine," *Journal for Eighteenth-Century Studies* 46, no. 1 (2023): 41–57.
6. Laqueur, "Orgasm." Also see Thomas Laqueur, *Making Sex: Body and Gender from the Greeks to Freud* (Cambridge, MA: Harvard University Press, 1992).

7. King's most recent work, a book-length examination of Laqueur's *Making Sex*, presents further evidence from the classical world and early modern Europe that emphasizes the failure of the one-sex model to account for the discursive complexities at the time. Considering Hippocratic gynecology in her argument, King offers a more nuanced analysis of the sexual politics of body models. Helen King, *The One-Sex Body on Trial: The Classical and Early Modern Evidence* (Burlington, VT: Ashgate, 2013).
8. Thomas Keymer, introduction to *"Joseph Andrews" and "Shamela,"* ed. Douglas Brooks-Davies (Oxford: Oxford University Press, 1999), xi.
9. Thomas Lockwood, "Shamela," *The Cambridge Companion to Henry Fielding*, ed. Claude Rawson (Cambridge: Cambridge University Press, 2007), 39.
10. "Anti-Pamelists" read Pamela as a self-interested, materialistic manipulator, especially with her fascination and cataloguing of material goods. Catherine Ingrassia, introduction to *Anti-Pamela and Shamela*, ed. Catherine Ingrassia (Peterborough, ON: Broadview, 2004), 15.
11. Nancy Armstrong, *Desire and Domestic Fiction: A Political History of the Novel* (New York: Oxford University Press, 1987), 31.
12. N. Armstrong, *Desire and Domestic Fiction*, 118.
13. Cissie Fairchilds, *Domestic Enemies: Servants and Their Masters in Old Regime France* (Baltimore: Johns Hopkins University Press, 2019), 174.
14. Fairchilds, *Domestic Enemies*, 101.
15. Georg Lukács, *The Historical Novel*, trans. Hannah Mitchell and Stanley Mitchell (London: Merlin, 1962), 94.
16. Bruce Robbins, *The Servant's Hand : English Fiction from Below* (New York: Columbia University Press, 1986), 75.
17. Following Fielding's *Shamela* was a flood of more or less hostile responses in print to *Pamela*. Cf. Thomas Keymer and Peter Sabor, eds., *The Pamela Controversy: Criticisms and Adaptations of Samuel Richardson's "Pamela," 1740–1750*, 6 vols. (London: Pickering and Chatto, 2001).
18. Henry Fielding, *An Apology for the Life of Mrs. Shamela Andrews* (1741), ed. Douglas Brooks-Davies (Oxford: Oxford University Press, 1999), 324.
19. Ingrassia, introduction to *Anti-Pamela and Shamela*, 9.
20. Martin Battestin, *The Moral Basis of Fielding's Art: A Study of "Joseph Andrews"* (Middletown, CT: Wesleyan University Press, 1959), 8–10.
21. Michael McKeon, *Origins of the English Novel, 1600–1740* (Baltimore: Johns Hopkins University Press, 2002), 396.
22. Robbins, *Servant's Hand*, 60.
23. According to a midcentury tract, the lines between domestic work and prostitution were blurry: "The Town being over stock'd with *Harlots*, is entirely owing to those Numbers of *Women-Servants*, incessantly pouring into it from all Corners of the Universe, and those Debaucheries practis'd upon 'em in almost all the Families that entertain them: *Masters, Footmen, Journeymen, Lodgers, Apprentices, &c.* are for ever attempting to corrupt. . . . Many of them are as restless as new *Equipage*, running from Place to Place, from Bawdy-House to Service, and from Service to Bawdy-House again; . . . So that in Effect, they neither make good Whores, good Wives, or good Servants, and this is one of the chief Reasons why our Streets swarm with Strumpets." Quoted in Michael McKeon, *The Secret History of Domesticity: Public, Private, and the Division of Knowledge* (Baltimore: Johns Hopkins University Press, 2005), 194–195.
24. Freind, *Emmenologia*, 22.
25. John Leake, *Medical instructions towards the prevention and cure of chronic diseases peculiar to women; In which, their Nature is fully explained, and their Treatment, by Regimen and simple Medicines, clearly laid down, divested of the Terms of Art, for the use of those affected with such Diseases, as well as the Medical Reader* (London: R. Baldwin, 1781).
26. Alexandra Lord, "'The Great Arcana of the Deity': Menstruation and Menstrual Disorders in Eighteenth-Century British Thought," *Bulletin of the History of Medicine* 73 (1999): 43.

27. Lord, "Great Arcana of the Deity," 58.
28. Freind, *Emmenologia*, 110.
29. Prior to the implementation of clinical methodologies of precision, experimentation, and data collection, some midwives and male medical practitioners believed that any periodic discharge of bodily fluid, such as hemorrhoids, bleeding sores, or even semen or urine, could be defined in terms of the menses. Lord, "Great Arcana of the Deity," 41–42.
30. Lord, "Great Arcana of the Deity," 70.
31. Ula Lukszo Klein, "Eighteenth-Century Female Cross-Dressers and Their Beards," *Journal for Early Modern Cultural Studies* 16, no. 4 (2016): 121.
32. Jacques-Antoine Dulaure, *Pogonologia; or, A Philosophical and Historical Essay on Beards. Translated from the French* (Exeter, 1786), 52.
33. Scholarly, elite women have also been assigned as "bearded:" For example, Immanuel Kant claimed that "a woman who has a head full of Greek, like Madame Dacier, or one who engages in debate about the intricacies of mechanics, like the Marquise du Chatelet, might just as well have a beard; for that expresses in a more recognizable form the profundity for which she strives." Immanuel Kant, *Beobachtungen uber das Gefuhl des Schonen und Erhabenen*, in *Kants Werke*, ed. Wilhelm Dilthey (Berlin, 1900–1919), 229–230.
34. Thomas Lockwood, "Theatrical Fielding," *Studies in the Literary Imagination* 32 (1999): 107–110; Lockwood, "Fielding from Stage to Page," in *Henry Fielding: Novelist, Playwright, Journalist, Magistrate (1707–1754)*, ed. Claude Rawson (Newark: Delaware University Press, 2008), 21–39.
35. Alexander Pope, *An Epistle to a Lady* (1735), in *Selected Poetry*, ed. Pat Rogers (Oxford: Oxford University Press, 1998), 106.
36. Freind, *Emmenologia*, 71.
37. Freind, *Emmenologia*, 91–92.
38. John Donne, *The Complete English Poems* (London: Penguin, 2004), ebook.
39. *The Spectator*, vol. 5 (London: Printed for S. Buckley and J. Tonson, 1713), 413, Eighteenth Century Collections Online.
40. Ruth Yeazell, *Fictions of Modesty: Women and Courtship in the English Novel* (Chicago: University of Chicago Press, 1991), 74.
41. Allen Michie, *Richardson and Fielding: The Dynamics of a Critical Rivalry* (Lewisburg, PA: Bucknell University Press, 1999).
42. Elizabeth Heckendorn Cook, *Epistolary Bodies: Gender and Genre in the Eighteenth-Century Republic of Letters* (Stanford, CA: Stanford University Press, 1996), 6.
43. Cook, *Epistolary Bodies*, 8.
44. Nicola Watson, *Revolution and the Form of the British Novel, 1790–1825: Intercepted Letters, Interrupted Seductions* (Oxford, UK: Clarendon, 1994), 2, 4.
45. Samuel Richardson, *Pamela; or, With Virtue Rewarded* (1740), ed. T. C. Duncan Eaves and Ben D. Kimpel (Boston: Houghton Mifflin, 1971), 39–40.
46. Jessica L. Leiman, "'Booby's Fruitless Operations': The Crisis of Male Authority in Richardson's *Pamela*," *Eighteenth-Century Fiction* 22, no. 2 (2009–2010): 235.
47. On female writing and immodesty, see Patricia Crawford, "Women's Published Writings 1600–1700," in *Women in English Society 1500–1800*, ed. Mary Prior (London: Methuen, 1985), 211–282; Janet Todd, *The Sign of Angellica: Women, Writing and Fiction, 1660–1800* (New York: Columbia University Press, 1989); Jeslyn Medoff, "The Daughters of Behn and the Problem of Reputation," in *Women, Writing, History 1640–1740*, ed. Isobel Grundy and Susan Wiseman (Athens: University of Georgia Press, 1992), and Catherine Gallagher, *Nobody's Story: The Vanishing Acts of Women Writers in the Marketplace, 1670–1820* (Berkeley: University of California Press, 1994).
48. Quoted in Wolfgang Zach, "Mrs Aubin and Richardson's Earliest Literary Manifesto (1739)," *English Studies* 62 (1981): 283.
49. Elizabeth Carter, *Letters from Mrs. Elizabeth Carter to Mrs. Montagu, 1755–1800*, ed. Montagu Pennington (London: F. C. and J. Rivington, 1817), 373.

50. Claudio Guillén, *Literature as System: Essays toward the Theory of Literary History* (Princeton, NJ: Princeton University Press, 2015), 81–82, 93.
51. Scarlet Bowen, "'A Sawce-box and Boldface Indeed': Refiguring the Female Servant in the Pamela-Antipamela Debate," *Studies in Eighteenth-Century Culture* 28 (1999), 270.
52. Bowen, "Sawce-box and Boldface Indeed," 259.
53. Terry Castle, *Clarissa's Cyphers: Meaning and Disruption in Richardson's "Clarissa"* (Ithaca, NY: Cornell University Press, 1982), 169.
54. Armstrong, *Desire and Domestic Fiction*, 138.
55. Jocelyn Harris, *Samuel Richardson* (Cambridge: Cambridge University Press, 1987), 33.
56. *A Present for Servants: From Their Ministers, Masters, or Other Friends*, 2nd ed. (London: J. Downing, 1710), 14.
57. Armstrong, *Desire and Domestic Fiction*, 112, 113.
58. Robert D. Spector, *Smollett's Women: A Study in Eighteenth-Century Masculine Sensibility* (Westport, CT: Greenwood, 1994), 171.
59. Jeremy Lewis, introduction to *Humphry Clinker*, by Tobias Smollett (London: Penguin Classics, 2008), xxiv.
60. Esther K. Sheldon, "What's an Impfiddle?," *American Speech*, 50, nos. 1–2 (1975): 138, 140.
61. Austin Dobson, *Eighteenth-Century Vignettes*: *Second Series* (London: Chatto and Windus, 1894), 133. Dobson points specifically to Win's substitution of "grease" for divine grace.
62. James L. Thorson, preface to *The Expedition of Humphry Clinker*, by Tobias Smollett (New York: Norton, 1983), xiv; Jerry Beasley, *Tobias Smollett: Novelist* (Athens: University of Georgia Press, 1998), 10–11.
63. George S. Rousseau, "Matt Bramble and the Sulphur Controversy in the Eighteenth Century," *Journal of the History of Ideas* 28 (1967): 577–599; David Weed, "Sentimental Misogyny and Medicine in *Humphry Clinker*," *Studies in English Literature, 1500–1900*, 37, no. 3 (1997): 615–636.
64. Aileen Douglas, *Uneasy Sensations: Smollett and the Body* (Chicago: University of Chicago Press, 1994).
65. John McAllister, "Smollett's Semiology of Emotions: The Symptomology of the Passions and Affections in *Roderick Random* and *Peregrine Pickle*," *English Studies in Canada* 14 (1988): 286–295; McAllister, "Smollett's Use of Medical Theory: *Roderick Random* and *Peregrine Pickle*," *Mosaic* 22 (1989): 121–130.
66. Tobias Smollett, *The Expedition of Humphry Clinker* (1771), ed. James L. Thorson (New York: Norton, 1983), 146. Subsequent references are to this edition and are cited parenthetically in the text.
67. Barbara Duden, *The Woman beneath the Skin: A Doctor's Patients in Seventeenth-Century Germany* (Cambridge: Cambridge University Press, 1991).
68. Herman Boerhaave, *Boerhaave's Aphorisms: Concerning the Knowledge and Cure of Diseases.* Translated from the last edition printed in Latin at Leyden, 1728 (London: W. Innys and C. Hitch, 1728), 312.
69. Boerhaave, *Boerhaave's Aphorisms*, 316.
70. Séverine Pilloud and Micheline Louis-Courvoisier, "The Intimate Experience of the Body in the Eighteenth Century: Between Interiority and Exteriority," *Medical History* 47, no. 4 (2003): 471.
71. Bakhtin, *Rabelais and His World*, 62.
72. Richard Steele, *The Tatler*, ed. Donald F. Bond (London: Oxford University Press, 1987); Richard Steele and Joseph Addison, *The Spectator*, ed. Donald F. Bond (London: Oxford University Press, 1965); Daniel Defoe, *Compleat English Gentleman*, ed. Karl D. Bülbring (Edinburgh: Ballantyne, 2006); Jonathan Swift, *A Proposal for Correcting, Improving and Ascertaining the English Tongue* (London: Tooke, 1712).
73. Thomas Sheridan, *Dissertation on the Causes of the Difficulties, Which Occur, in Learning of the English Tongue* (London: R. and J. Dodsley, 1762), 3.
74. Richman, "Other King's Speech," 284.

75. Richman, "Other King's Speech," 284.
76. Lennard J. Davis, *Bending Over Backwards: Disability, Dismodernism, and Other Difficult Positions* (New York: New York University Press, 2002), 107.
77. Joshua, "Disability and Deformity," 47.
78. Deutsch and Nussbaum, introduction to *"Defects,"* 11.
79. Lennard J. Davis, "Dr. Johnson, Amelia, and the Discourse of Disability in the Eighteenth Century, in Deutsch and Nussbaum, *"Defects,"* 57, 56.
80. Bakhtin, *Rabelais and His World*, 10.
81. Freind, *Emmenologia*, i.
82. J. Paul Hunter, *Before Novels: The Cultural Contexts of Eighteenth-Century English Fiction* (New York: Norton, 1990); Fergus, "Provincial Servants' Reading."
83. Since the sixteenth and seventeenth centuries, reformers and benefactors showered the underclass with sermons and pamphlets, disseminating the message that worldly and heavenly rewards lay in wait for laboring families who were meek and did what they were told. Charities such as the Society for the Promotion of Christian Knowledge (1699) and the Society for Distributing Religious Tracts Among the Poor (1782) issued tracts of Christian truth. Roy Porter, *English Society in the Eighteenth Century* (London: Penguin, 1991), 295.
84. Frank, *Common Ground*, 47.
85. Anthony Ashley Cooper, Third Earl of Shaftesbury, *Characteristics of Men, Manners, Opinions, Times with a Collection of Letters by the Right Honorable Anthony Shaftesbury*, vol. 3 (Basil: Tourneisen and Legrand, 1790), 149–150.
86. See Dickie, *Cruelty and Laughter*; and Roger Lund, "Laughing at Cripples: Ridicule, Deformity and the Argument from Design," *Eighteenth Century Studies* 39, no. 1 (2005): 91–114.
87. Simon Dickie, "Hilarity and Pitilessness in the Mid-Eighteenth Century: English Jestbook Humor," *Eighteenth-Century Studies* 37, no. 1 (2003): 16.
88. Tobias Smollett, *The Adventures of Ferdinand Count Fathom* (1753), ed. Jerry C. Beasley (Athens: University of Georgia Press, 2014), 43.
89. "'Weep 'Weep!'": History of Chimney Sweeps," *History Magazine* 12, no. 6 (2011): 42–44.
90. Mikhail Bakhtin, *The Dialogic Imagination: Four Essays*, ed. Michael Holquist, trans. Caryl Emerson and Michael Holquist (Austin: University of Texas Press, 1981), 270.
91. Frank Donahue, "Colonizing Readers: Review Criticism and the Formation of a Reading Public," in *The Consumption of Culture: Image, Object, Text*, ed. Ann Bermingham and John Brewer (London: Routledge, 1995), 57–74.
92. Naomi Tadmor, "'In the Even My Wife Read to Me': Women, Reading, and Household Life in the Eighteenth Century," in *The Practice and Representation of Reading in England*, ed. James Raven, Helen Small, and Naomi Tadmor (Cambridge: Cambridge University Press, 1996), 167.
93. James Raven, "From Promotion to Proscription: Arrangements for Reading and Eighteenth-Century Libraries," in Raven et al., *Practice and Representation*, 176.
94. Fergus, "Provincial Servants' Reading," 202–205.
95. John Brewer, *The Pleasures of the Imagination: English Culture in the Eighteenth Century* (New York: Farrar, Straus and Giroux, 1997), 187.
96. Adam Fox, "Popular Verses and Their Readership in the Early Seventeenth0 Century," in Raven et al., *Practice and Representation*, 125–137.
97. "Reading community" is a development of Stanley Fish's work on "interpretive communities," a group of readers who bring particular "interpretative strategies" to a text. Stanley Fish, *Is There a Text in This Class? The Authority of Interpretive Communities* (Cambridge, MA: Harvard University Press, 1980). Kate Jackson defines the development of reading communities as "categories of readers linked together by a common experience or expectation of reading and by common social, political, ideological or cultural objectives or bonds rather than by physical proximity." Kate Jackson, *George Newnes and the New Journalism in Britain 1880–1910: Culture and Profit* (Aldershot, UK: Ashgate, 2001), 11.
98. Bakhtin, *Rabelais and His World*, 11.

## CHAPTER 2 — HYSTERICAL LANGUAGE AND DESIRING WOMEN IN HENRY FIELDING'S *JOSEPH ANDREWS* (1742) AND *TOM JONES* (1749)

1. Nina Prytula, "'Great-Breasted and Fierce': Fielding's Amazonian Heroines," *Eighteenth Century Studies* 35, no. 2 (2002): 176.
2. Many scholars have turned to *The Female Husband* to examine the contradictions in Fielding's ideologies on gender. See Emma Donoghue, *Passions between Women: British Lesbian Culture 1668–1801* (New York: Harper Perennial, 1996), 73–80; Jack Halberstam, *Female Masculinity* (Durham, NC: Duke University Press, 2018), 50–53, 67; and Sal Nicolazzo, "Henry Fielding's *The Female Husband* and the Sexuality of Vagrancy," *The Eighteenth Century* 55, no. 4 (2014): 335–353.
3. Henry Fielding, *Tom Jones*, ed. John Bender and Simon Stern (1749; Oxford: Oxford University Press, 1996), 543. Subsequent references are to this edition and are cited parenthetically in the text.
4. Carolyn Merchant, *The Death of Nature: Women, Ecology, and the Scientific Revolution* (San Francisco: Harper and Row, 1980); Keller, *Reflections on Gender and Science.*
5. Tita Chico, *The Experimental Imagination: Literary Knowledge and Science in the British Enlightenment* (Stanford, CA: Stanford University Press, 2018), 12.
6. Recent works on emotion in the long eighteenth century include Thomas Dixon, *From Passions to Emotions: The Creation of a Secular Psychological Category* (Cambridge: Cambridge University Press, 2003); Heather Kerr, David Lemmings, and Robert Phiddian, eds., *Passions, Sympathy and Print Culture: Public Opinion and Emotional Authenticity in Eighteenth-Century Britain* (New York: Palgrave Macmillan, 2016); Susan Broomhall, ed., *Spaces for Feeling: Gender, Affect, and Sociability in Britain, 1650–1850* (New York: Routledge, 2015); and James Noggle, *Unfelt: The Language of Affect in the British Enlightenment* (Ithaca, NY: Cornell University Press, 2020).
7. Dixon, *From Passions to Emotions*, 72.
8. Rebecca Tierney-Hynes discusses the link between the development of the novel and philosophical discourse in *Novel Minds: Philosophers and Romance Readers, 1680–1740* (Basingstoke, UK: Palgrave Macmillan, 2012).
9. Heather Meek, "Of Wandering Wombs and Wrongs of Women: Evolving Conceptions of Hysteria in the Age of Reason," *ECS* 35, nos. 2–3 (2009): 118.
10. Sabine Arnaud, *On Hysteria: The Invention of a Medical Category between 1670 and 1820* (Chicago: University of Chicago Press, 2015), 69.
11. Guenter Risse, "Hysteria at the Edinburgh Infirmary: The Construction and Treatment of a Disease, 1770–1800," *Medical History* 32, no. 1 (1988): 17.
12. Glen Colburn, "Struggling Manfully through Henry Fielding's *Amelia*: Hysteria, Medicine, and the Novel in Eighteenth-Century England," *Studies in Eighteenth-Century Culture* 26 (1997): 98.
13. See Robert Alter, *Fielding and the Nature of the Novel* (Cambridge, MA: Harvard University Press, 1968); Gary Gautier, "Marriage and Family in Fielding's Fiction," *Studies in the Novel* 27, no. 2 (1995): 111–128; John J. Richetti, "Voice and Gender in Eighteenth-Century Fiction: Haywood to Burney," *Studies in the Novel* 19, no. 3 (1987): 263–272; Ronald Paulson, *The Life of Henry Fielding: A Critical Biography* (Oxford, UK: Blackwell, 2000).
14. Paul Kelleher, *Making Love: Sentiment and Sexuality in Eighteenth-Century British Literature* (Lewisburg, PA: Bucknell University Press, 2015).
15. Tiffany Potter, *Honest Sins: Georgian Libertinism and the Plays and Novels of Henry Fielding* (Montreal: McGill-Queen's University Press, 1999), 23.
16. Potter, *Honest Sins*, 24.
17. James Boswell, *Life of Johnson*, ed. George B. Hill, 4 vols. (Oxford: Oxford University Press, 1994), 2:48–49.
18. Thomas Sydenham, *Epistle to Dr. Cole*, in *The Works of Thomas Sydenham*, trans. R. D. Latham (London: Sydenham Society, 1852), 74.

19. Sydenham, *Epistle to Dr. Cole*, 79.
20. Sydenham, *Epistle to Dr. Cole*, 90.
21. Richard Blackmore, *A Treatise of the Spleen and Vapours; or Hypochondriacal and Hysterical Affections. With Three Discourses on the Nature and Cure of the Cholick, Melancholy, and Palsies* (London: Pemberton, 1726), 96.
22. Jordanova, *Sexual Visions*, 2.
23. Eliza Haywood, *The Female Spectator* (1744–1746), in *Selected Works of Eliza Haywood*, ed. Kathryn R. King and Alexander Pettit (London: Pickering and Chatto, 2001), 360.
24. For more on Fielding and Haywood's professional relationship, see Kathryn R. King, "Henry and Eliza: Feudlings or Friends?," in *Henry Fielding in Our Time: Papers Presented at the Tercentenary Conference*, ed. J. A. Downie (Newcastle upon Tyne: Cambridge Scholars, 2008), 215–231.
25. William Empson, "Tom Jones," *Kenyon Review* 20 (1958): 217–259; reprinted in *Fielding: A Collection of Critical Essays*, ed. Ronald Paulson (Englewood Cliffs, NJ: Prentice Hall, 1962), 124–126.
26. Henry Fielding, *Joseph Andrews* (1741), ed. Douglas Brooks-Davies (Oxford: Oxford University Press, 1999), 34. Subsequent references are to this edition and are cited parenthetically in the text.
27. James Mackenzie, *The History of Health* (Edinburgh: William Gordon, 1758), 388.
28. Eliza Haywood, *Fantomina and Other Works*, ed. Alexander Pettit, Margaret Case Croskery, and Anna C. Patchias (Peterborough, ON: Broadview, 2004), 63.
29. Paulson, *Life of Henry Fielding*, 147–148.
30. Many critics have observed that examining depictions of emotion in eighteenth-century literature offers a space to understand early modern persons. See Alan T. McKenzie, *Certain Lively Episodes: The Articulation of Passion in Eighteenth-Century Prose* (Athens: University of Georgia Press, 1990); and Tierney-Hynes, *Novel Minds*.
31. For more on how writers and medical thinkers visualized and explained the operations of the mind and the body, see Jess Keiser, *Nervous Fictions: Literary Form and the Enlightenment Origins of Neuroscience* (Charlottesville: University of Virginia Press, 2020).
32. Stephen Ahern, "Nothing More than Feelings? Affect Theory Reads the Age of Sensibility," *Eighteenth Century: Theory and Interpretation* 58, no. 3 (2017): 283.
33. Ahern, "Nothing More than Feelings?," 284.
34. Stephen Ahern, *Affected Sensibilities: Romantic Excess and the Genealogy of the Novel* (New York: AMS Press, 2007), 27.
35. Ahern, *Affected Sensibilities*, 41.
36. Ahern, *Affected Sensibilities*, 81.
37. Quoted in Ahern, *Affected Sensibilities*, 79.
38. Ahern, *Affected Sensibilities*, 79.
39. Andrew Scull, *Hysteria: The Biography* (Oxford: Oxford University Press, 2009).
40. William Cullen, *First Lines of the Practice of Physic*, vol. 2 (Edinburgh: Reid and Bathgate, 1784), 153.
41. Edward Hare, "The History of 'Nervous Disorders' from 1600 to 1840, and a Comparison with Modern Views," *British Journal of Psychiatry* 159, no. 1 (1991): 41.
42. Quoted in Lindemann, *Medicine and Society*, 106.
43. Freind, *Emmenologia*, 18.
44. Meek, "Of Wandering Wombs," 108.
45. Robert Whytt, *Observations on the Nature, Causes, and Cure of Those Disorders Which Are Commonly Called Nervous, Hypochondriac, or Hysteric. To Which Are Prefixed Some Remarks on the Sympathy of the Nerves, 1764* (London : T. Maiden, 1797), 6.
46. Aleksondra Hultquist, "Eliza Haywood's Progress through the Passions," in *Passions, Sympathy and Print Culture: Public Opinion and Emotional Authenticity in Eighteenth-*

*Century Britain*, ed. Heather Kerr, David Lemmings, and Robert Phiddian (New York: Palgrave Macmillan, 2016), 88.

47. Eliza Haywood, *Love in Excess; or, The Fatal Enquiry*, ed. David Oakleaf (Peterborough, ON: Broadview, 2000), 116.
48. Blackmore, *Treatise of the Spleen and Vapours*, 35.
49. Hultquist, "Eliza Haywood's Progress," 98.
50. For more on the theory of countervailing passions in eighteenth-century philosophy, see A. O. Hirschman, *The Passions and the Interests* (Princeton, NJ: Princeton University Press, 1977).
51. Potter, *Honest Sins*, 94.
52. Paul Baines, "Joseph Andrews," in *The Cambridge Companion to Henry Fielding*, ed. Claude Rawson (Cambridge: Cambridge University Press, 2007), 57.
53. Tiffany Potter, "'A Certain Sign That He Is One of Use': *Clarissa*'s Other Libertines," *Eighteenth-Century Fiction* 11, no. 4 (1999): 405.
54. Potter, *Honest Sins*, 125.
55. Haywood, *Love in Excess*, 120.
56. Richard Mead, *Medical Precepts and Cautions* (London: 1751), 280.
57. John Ball, *The Female Physician; or, Every Woman Her Own Doctor* (London, 1777), 11.
58. Daniel Defoe, *Conjugal Lewdness; or, Matrimonial Whoredom. A Treatise concerning the Use and Abuse of the Marriage Bed* (1727; repr., Gainesville, FL: Scholars' Facsimiles and Reprints, 1967), 123, 133.
59. Quoted in Angus McLaren, *Reproductive Rituals: The Perception of Fertility in England from the Sixteenth Century to the Nineteenth Century* (New York: Methuen, 1984), 22.
60. Terry Castle, *Masquerades and Civilization: The Carnivalesque in Eighteenth-Century Culture and Fiction* (Stanford, CA: Stanford University Press, 1986), 78.
61. Eliza Haywood, *The Injur'd Husband; or, The Mistaken Resentment and Lasselia; or, The Self-Abandon'd* (1722), ed. Jerry C. Beasley (Lexington: University Press of Kentucky, 1999); Haywood, *The Perplex'd Dutchess; or, Treachery Rewarded* (1727); Haywood, *The Force of Nature; or, The Lucky Disappointment* (1724).
62. Andrea Austin, "Shooting Blanks: Potency, Parody, and Eliza Haywood's *The History of Miss Betsy Thoughtless*," in *The Passionate Fictions of Eliza Haywood*, ed. Kirsten T. Saxton and Rebecca P. Bocchicchio (Lexington: University Press of Kentucky, 2000), 271.
63. Samuel Richardson, *Clarissa; or, The History of a Young Lady* (1748; repr., London: Penguin, 1986), 3.
64. Henry Fielding to Sarah Fielding, October 15, 1748, in *Correspondence of Henry and Sarah Fielding*, ed. Martin C. Battestin and Clive T. Probyn (Oxford, UK: Clarendon, 1993), 70–74.
65. Ros Ballaster, *Seductive Forms: Women's Amatory Fiction from 1684 to 1740* (Oxford: Oxford University Press, 1992), 179.
66. Castle, *Masquerades and Civilization*, 43.
67. Colburn, "Struggling Manfully," 89.
68. Blackmore, *Treatise of the Spleen and Vapours*, 107.
69. Nicholas Robinson, *A New System of the Spleen, Vapours, and Hypochondriack Melancholy* (London: Bettesworth, 1729), 214.
70. Eliza Fowler Haywood, *Life's Progress through the Passions: or, the Adventures of Natura* (London: T. Gardner, 1748), 18.
71. Cook, *Epistolary Bodies*, 8.
72. Barbara Maria Zaczek, *Censored Sentiments: Letters and Censorship in Epistolary Novels and Conduct Material* (Newark: University of Delaware Press, 1997).
73. Ahern, *Affected Sensibilities*, 83.
74. Richard Terry, "'P.S.': The Dangerous Logic of the Postscript in Eighteenth-Century Literature," *Modern Language Review* 109, no. 1 (2014): 42.

75. Terry, "P.S.," 43.
76. Ahern, *Affected Sensibilities*, 84.
77. [Sarah Chapone], *The Hardship of the English Laws in Relation to Wives* (London: W. Boyer, 1735), 2.
78. Meek, "Of Wandering Wombs," 119–120.
79. Haywood, *Life's Progress*, 168–169.
80. Haywood, *Life's Progress*, 185.
81. Simon Dickie, *Cruelty and Laughter: Forgotten Comic Literature and the Unsentimental Eighteenth Century* (Chicago: University of Chicago Press, 2014), 220–221.
82. Sharon Harrow, "Having Text: Desire and Language in Haywood's *Love in Excess* and *The Distressed Orphan*," *Eighteenth Century Fiction* 22, no. 2 (2009): 295.
83. Zaczek, *Censored Sentiments*, 13.
84. Jerry C. Beasley, introduction to Haywood, *Injur'd Husband*, xxv, ix–xxxviii.
85. Haywood, *Injur'd Husband*, 100.
86. Angela J. Smallwood, *Fielding and the Woman Question* (New York: St. Martin's, 1989).
87. *Grub Street Journal*, June 1, 1732, in *Henry Fielding: The Critical Heritage*, ed. Ronald Paulson and Thomas Lockwood (London: Routledge, 1969), 39–43.
88. Baines, "Joseph Andrews," 56.

## CHAPTER 3 — THE MATERNAL BODY AND OBSTETRIC AUTHORITY IN LAURENCE STERNE'S *TRISTRAM SHANDY* (1759) AND TOBIAS SMOLLETT'S *PEREGRINE PICKLE* (1751)

1. Marilyn Francus, "The Monstrous Mother: Reproductive Anxiety in Swift and Pope," *ELH* 61, no. 4 (1994): 829.
2. Susan Gubar, "The Female Monster in Augustan Satire," *Signs* 3 (1977): 380–394.
3. Luce Irigaray, "This Sex Which Is Not One," in *This Sex Which Is Not One* (Ithaca, NY: Cornell University Press, 1985), 26.
4. Bakhtin, *Rabelais and His World*, 62.
5. William Harvey, *Anatomic Exercises on the Generation of Animals*, in *The Works of William Harvey*, trans. Robert Willis (London: Sydenham Society, 1847), 271.
6. Laurence Sterne, *The Life and Opinions of Tristram Shandy*, ed. Ian Campbell Ross (Oxford: Oxford University Press, 2000), 315. Subsequent references are to this edition and are cited parenthetically in the text.
7. William Sermon, *The Ladies Companion; or, The English Midwife* (London: Edward Thomas, 1671), B1V.
8. Brudenell Exton, *A New and General System of Midwifery in Four Parts* (London: W. Owen, 1753), 19.
9. E. Ann Kaplan, *Motherhood and Representation: The Mother in Popular Culture and Melodrama* (London: Routledge, 1992), 19.
10. Ruth Perry, "Words for Sex: The Verbal Sexual Continuum in *Tristram Shandy*," *Studies in the Novel* 20 (1988): 34, 37, 42; Leigh A. Ehlers, "Mrs. Shandy's 'Lint and Basilicon': The Importance of Women in *Tristram Shandy*," *South Atlantic Review* 46 (1981): 61–73; Ruth Faurot, "Mrs. Shandy Observed," *Studies in English Literature* 10 (1970): 579–589.
11. Francus, "Monstrous Mother," 844.
12. Naomi Tadmor has written on the expanded definition of family in the seventeenth and eighteenth centuries to include servants and apprentices, signifying close kinship beyond blood relations. Naomi Tadmor, "The Concept of the Household-Family in Eighteenth-Century England," *Past and Present* 151 (1995): 111–140.
13. Elizabeth Nihell, *A Treatise on the Art of Midwifery* (London: A. Morley 1760), 15.
14. Nihell, *Treatise on the Art of Midwifery*, 98–99.
15. John Locke, *Two Treatises of Government* (1689), ed. Peter Laslett (New York: New American Library, 1965), § 6.

16. Susan C. Greenfield, "Aborting the 'Mother Plot': Politics and Generation in *Absolom and Achitophel*," in *Inventing Maternity: Politics, Science, and Literature, 1650–1865*, ed. Susan C. Greenfield and Carol Barash (Lexington: University Press of Kentucky, 1999), 89.
17. Thomas Hobbes, *De Cive: The English Version* (1642), ed. Howard Warrender (Oxford, UK: Clarendon, 1983), 123; Hobbes, *Leviathan* (1651), ed. C. B. Macpherson (Harmondsworth, UK: Penguin Books, 1985), 253–254.
18. Robert Filmer, *Patriarcha and Other Writings*, ed. Johann P. Sommerville (Cambridge: Cambridge University Press, 1991), 1, 10, 11–12.
19. Filmer, *Patriarcha*, 192.
20. Ludmilla Jordanova, "Interrogating the Concept of Reproduction in the Eighteenth Century," in *Conceiving the New World Order: the Global Politics of Reproduction*, ed. Faye Ginsburg and Rayna Rapp (Berkeley: University of California Press, 1995), 371–374.
21. Judith Schneid Lewis, *In the Family Way: Childbearing in the British Aristocracy, 1760–1860* (New Brunswick, NJ: Rutgers University Press, 1986).
22. Juliet McMaster, "Walter Shandy, Sterne, and Gender: A Feminist Foray," in *Critical Essays on Laurence Sterne*, ed. Melvyn New (New York: G. K. Hall, 1998), 205.
23. Mark Breitenberg, *Anxious Masculinity in Early Modern England* (Cambridge: Cambridge University Press, 1996), 2.
24. Aristotle, *Generation of Animals*, trans. A. Platt, in *The Complete Works of Aristotle*, ed. J. Barnes (Princeton: Princeton University Press, 1984), 729.b.15ff.
25. Quoted in Laqueur, *Making Sex*, 30.
26. Eve Keller, "Making Up for Losses: The Workings of Gender in William Harvey's *de Generatione animalium*," in *Inventing Maternity: Politics, Science, and Literature, 1650–1865*, ed. Susan C. Greenfield and Carol Barash (Lexington: University Press of Kentucky, 1999), 39.
27. Harvey, *Anatomic Exercises*, 575.
28. Harvey, *Anatomic Exercises*, 322.
29. Harvey, *Anatomic Exercises*, 322.
30. Keller, "Making Up for Losses," 45.
31. Keller, "Making Up for Losses," 48.
32. For more on Harvey's theory of generation, particularly as it relates to questions of gender and subjectivity, see Keller, "Making Up for Losses."
33. Nathaniel Highmore, *The History of Generation* (London: John Martin, 1651), 86.
34. Felicity A. Nussbaum, "'Savage' Mothers: Narratives of Maternity in the Mid-Eighteenth Century," *Cultural Critique*, no. 20 (1991): 126.
35. Juliet McMaster, "'Uncrystallized Flesh and Blood': The Body in *Tristram Shandy*," *Eighteenth-Century Fiction* 2, no. 3 (1990): 212.
36. Judith Hawley notes that "the health of both Tristram's person . . . depends upon that first act of conception." She describes Walter as "unashamedly 'animalculist.'" According to traducianism, Trismegistus's favored theory of conception, the father's semen not only gave a child his father's likeness but also gave him his soul. Eve Keller's study of the history of eighteenth-century embryology and its role in constructing early modern subjecthood explains preformation theory—a medical perspective similar to traducianism. Preformation asserts that the entire future organism's parts were formed prior to conception in the body of either of the parents. This means that the future baby could be theoretically identified in either the woman (the ovum) or the man (the animalcule in the sperm). Since preformation was the most common medical theory at the end of the century—with George Garden's, Rene de Graaf's, and Anton von Leeuwenhoek's discoveries contributing to its legitimacy in some way—it should be unsurprising that Walter's self-flagellation has medical grounds. Judith Hawley, "The Anatomy of *Tristram Shandy*," in *Literature and Medicine during the Eighteenth Century* (London: Routledge, 1993), 84, 88; Eve Keller, "Embryonic Individuals: The Rhetoric of Seventeenth-Century Embryology and the Construction of Early-Modern Identity," *Eighteenth-Century Studies* 33, no. 3 (2000): 331.

37. Erasmus Darwin, *Zoomonia; or, The Laws of Organic Life*, vol. 2 (London: J. Johnson, 1794), 520.
38. Breitenberg, *Anxious Masculinity*, 12.
39. See Jordanova, *Sexual Visions*.
40. Eve Keller writes that the characterization of a fetus as an infant or child contradicts ancient and even modern knowledge about early fetal status. In the legal arena of abortion cases, fetuses were not considered to be a whole human being before "quickening," or perceived fetal movement. Aristotle recognized the fetus to exist without being alive. For more, see Keller, "Embryonic Individuals."
41. *Arbor Vitae; or, The Natural History of the Tree of Life* (London: E. Hill, 1741), 12; [William Hewardine?], "The Marriage Morn," in *Hilaria, The Festive Board* (Printed for the Author, 1798), 9.
42. Merry E. Wiesner-Hanks, *Women and Gender in Early Modern Europe* (Cambridge: Cambridge University Press, 2000), 32.
43. John Armstrong, *The Oeconomy of Love: A Poetical Essay* (London: T. Cooper, 1736), 30.
44. *Arbor Vitae*, 4.
45. Paddy Strong-Cock [pseud.], *Teague-root Display'd: Being Some Useful and Important Discoveries Tending to Illustrate the Doctrine of Electricity* (London: W. Webb, 1746), 22.
46. *Arbor Vitae*, 4.
47. "A Short Sermon on Matrimony," *Lady's Magazine*, October 1783, 520.
48. *Secret History of Pandora's Box* (London: T. Cooper, 1742), 55.
49. Roy Porter, "'The Whole Secret of Health': Mind, Body and Medicine in *Tristram Shandy*," in *Nature Transfigured: Science and Literature, 1700–1900*, ed. John Christie and Sally Shuttleworth (Manchester, UK: Manchester University Press, 1989), 65.
50. Jacques Gélis, *History of Childbirth: Fertility, Pregnancy, and Birth in Early Modern Europe* (Boston: Northeastern University Press, 1991), 54.
51. Daniel Turner, *De morbis cutaneis* (London: R. Bonwicke 1723), 162.
52. D. Turner, *De morbis cutaneis*, 128.
53. James Augustus Blondel, *The Strength of Imagination in Pregnant Women* (London: J. Peele, 1727), preface.
54. Blondel, *Strength of Imagination*, 55.
55. Paul-Gabriel Boucé, "Imagination, Pregnant Women, and Monsters, in Eighteenth-Century England and France," in *Sexual Underworlds of the Enlightenment*, ed. G. S. Rousseau and Roy Porter (Chapel Hill: University of North Carolina Press, 1988), 99.
56. Julia Epstein, "The Pregnant Imagination, Women's Bodies, and Fetal Rights," in *Inventing Maternity: Politics, Science, and Literature, 1650–1865*, ed. Susan C. Greenfield and Carol Barash (Lexington: University Press of Kentucky, 1999), 121.
57. The eighteenth-century usage of "disability" referred to a ship or person transitively unfit for service, not necessarily bodily impairment. Chris Mounsey interrogates "disability" in binary terms, suggesting "variability" and "variable bodies" instead. Chris Mounsey, "Introduction: Variability: Beyond Sameness and Difference," in *The Idea of Disability in the Eighteenth Century*, ed. Chris Mounsey (Lewisburg, PA: Bucknell University Press, 1997), 1–27.
58. See Marie-Hélène Huet, *Monstrous Imagination* (Cambridge, MA: Harvard University Press, 1993), chaps. 1 and 2; and Ludmilla Jordanova, "Gender, Generation, and Science: William Hunter's Obstetrical Atlas," in *William Hunter and the Eighteenth-Century Medical World*, ed. W. F. Bynum and Roy Porter (Cambridge: Cambridge University Press, 1985), 402–412.
59. Claude Quillet, *La callipedie ou l'art d'avoir de beaux enfans* (Paris, 1749), Book III, 92.
60. Voltaire, "Influence," in *Philosophical Dictionary*, trans. Theodore Besterman (Harmondsworth, UK: Penguin, 1971).
61. John Maubray, *The Female Physician* (London: James Holland, 1724), 75–76.
62. Gélis, *History of Childbirth*, 154.

63. C.H.G Macafee, "The Obstetrical Aspects of *Tristram Shandy*," *Ulster Medical Journal* 19, no. 1 (1950): 17.
64. Macafee, "Obstetrical Aspects," 17.
65. Quoted in Herbert R. Spencer, *The History of British Midwifery: From 1650–1800* (New York: AMS Press, 1927), 36.
66. Maubray, *Female Physician*, 75–77.
67. François Mauriceau, *The Diseases of Women with Child and in Child-bed*, trans. Hugh Chamberlen (London: John Darby, 1683), 58, 65.
68. F. A. Deleurye, "Des passions de l'ame," in *Traité des accouchemens en faveur des élèves* (Paris, 1770), 93.
69. Alexander Hamilton, *A Treatise of Midwifery Comprehending the Management of Female Complaints, and the Treatment of Children in Early Infancy—Divested of Technical Terms and Abstruse Theories* (London: J. Murray; Edinburgh: Dickson, Creech, and Elliot, 1781), 161.
70. John Grigg, *Advice to the Female Sex in General, Particularly Those in a State of Pregnancy and Lying-In: The Complaints Incident to Their Respective Situations Are Specified, and Treatment Recommended, Agreeable to Modern Practice* (Bath, UK: S. Hazard, 1789), 117–118.
71. John Henry Mauclerc, *Dr. Blondel Confuted; or, The Ladies Vindicated, with Regard to the Power of Imagination in Pregnant Women: Together with a Circular and General Address to the Ladies, on This Occasion* (London: M. Cooper, 1747).
72. Claude E. Jones gives a brief history of Smollett's literary experience and friendships in medical circles in "An Essay on the External Use of Water, by Tobias Smollett," *Bulletin of the Institute of the History of Medicine* 3, no. 1 (1935): 31–82.
73. Beasley, *Tobias Smollett*, 80.
74. Tobias Smollett, *The Adventures of Peregrine Pickle* (1751), ed. James L. Clifford (Oxford: Oxford University Press, 1964), 53. Subsequent references are to this edition and are cited parenthetically in the text.
75. R. G. Collins reads Mrs. Pickle's desire for pineapples (a fruit medical professionals understood to be an abortion stimulant), her Spartan regimen for the baby Peregrine, and her fury at her first son's inheritance of the estate at his father's death as all signaling his illegitimacy. R. G. Collins, "The Hidden Bastard: A Question of Illegitimacy in Smollett's *Peregrine Pickle*," *PMLA* 94, no. 1 (1979): 91–105.
76. Francus, "Monstrous Mother," 851.
77. Nussbaum, "'Savage' Mothers," 127.
78. Richard Allestree, *The Ladies Calling*, 5th ed. (Oxford, UK, 1677), 201–213.
79. Toni Bowers, "'A Point of Conscience': Breastfeeding and Maternal Authority in *Pamela*, Part 2," in *Inventing Maternity: Politics, Science, and Literature, 1650–1865*, ed. Susan C. Greenfield and Carol Barash (Lexington: University Press of Kentucky, 1999), 145.
80. Ruth Perry, "Colonizing the Breast: Sexuality and Maternity in Eighteenth-Century England," *Journal of the History of Sexuality* 2, no. 2 (1991): 214.
81. John Locke, *Essay Concerning Human Understanding* (1689), ed. Peter H. Nidditch (Oxford, UK: Clarendon, 1975), 74.
82. Brian K. Nance, "Determining the Patient's Temperament: An Excursion into Seventeenth-Century Medical Semeiology," *Bulletin of the History of Medicine* 67, no. 3 (1993): 435.
83. William Buchan, *Domestic Medicin[e]; or, The Family Physician* (London: John Dunlap, 1772).
84. Buchan, *Domestic Medicin[e]*, 4. The father's responsibility mostly lies in how his infirmity or profligacy shapes an unhealthy or sickly child at conception, rather than raising or educating the child.
85. Maubray, *Female Physician*, 69.
86. William Stukeley, *Of the Spleen, Its Description and History* (London: Roberts, 1722), 50, 63.
87. Jerome Gaub, *De regimine mentis* (1747), trans. L. J. Rather (Berkeley: University of California Press, 1965): 34–114.

88. Richard Blackmore, "An Essay upon Wit," in *Essays Upon Several Subjects* (1716; repr., New York: Garland, 1971), 196–197.
89. Beasley, *Tobias Smollett*, 81.
90. Beasley, *Tobias Smollett*, 91–92.
91. John Skinner, *Constructions of Smollett: A Study of Genre and Gender* (Newark: University of Delaware Press, 1996), 74.
92. Simon Dickie, "Tobias Smollett and the Ramble Novel," in *The Oxford History of the Novel in English*, vol. 2, *English and British Fiction, 1750–1820*, ed. Peter Garside and Karen O'Brien (New York: Oxford University Press, 2015), 105.
93. Collins, "Hidden Bastard."
94. Beasley, *Tobias Smollett*, 81.
95. McAllister, "Smollett's Use of Medical Theory," 128, 129.
96. Tobias Smollett, *The Adventures of Roderick Random* (1748), ed. Paul-Gabriel Boucé (London: Oxford University Press, 1979), 435.
97. Linda Pollock, "Childbearing and Female Bonding in Early Modern England," *Social History* 22, no. 3 (1997): 286–306.
98. W. Johnstone, *William Smellie: The Master of British Midwifery* (Edinburgh: E & S Livingstone, 1952); L. Lewis Wall, "William Smellie (1697–1763), the Father of Scientific Obstetrics," *Medical Heritage* 2 (1986): 158–167.
99. Vicious pranks were a common characteristic in Smollett's novels, as well as in the popular "ramble" fiction of the 1750s and 1760s, and are cast as satiric episodes by critics. Dickie, "Tobias Smollett and the Ramble Novel," 98.
100. Jennifer Buckley, *Gender, Pregnancy and Power in Eighteenth-Century Literature: The Maternal Imagination* (Cham, Switzerland: Palgrave Macmillan, 2017), 84.
101. Mary Fissell, *Vernacular Bodies: The Politics of Reproduction in Early Modern England* (Oxford: Oxford University Press, 2004), 136.
102. Nicholas Culpeper, *A Directory for Midwives* (London: J. and A. Churchill, 1701), 2–3.
103. Culpeper, *Directory for Midwives*, 3.
104. Tobias Smollett, quoted in *Childbirth: Changing Ideas and Practices in Britain and America 1600 to the Present*, vol. 2, ed. Philip K. Wilson (New York: Garland, 1996), 47–48.
105. David Harley, "Provincial Midwives in England: Lancashire and Cheshire, 1660–1760," in *The Art of Midwifery: Early Modern Midwives in Europe*, ed. Hilary Marland (London: Routledge, 1993), 28.
106. Tobias Smollett, *A Complete History of England, Deduced from the Descent of Julius Cæsar, to the Treaty of Aix la Chapelle, 1748. Containing the Transactions of One Thousand Eight Hundred and Three Years. By T. Smollett, M.D. . . .* Vol. 1 (London: James Rivington and James Fletcher, 1757), Eighteenth Century Collections Online.
107. Harley, "Provincial Midwives," 38.
108. Harley, "Provincial Midwives," 42.
109. Harley, "Provincial Midwives," 41–42.
110. William Smellie, *A Treatise on the Theory and Practice of Midwifery* (London: Alexander Cleugh and M. Watson, 1790), 142.
111. Fissell, *Vernacular Bodies*, 142.
112. Culpeper, *Directory for Midwives*, 28.
113. Culpeper, *Directory for Midwives*, 278.
114. Culpeper, *Directory for Midwives*, 102.
115. G. S. Rousseau, "Pineapples, Pregnancy, Pica, and *Peregrine Pickle*," in *Tobias Smollett: Bicentennial Essays Presented to Lewis M. Knapp*, ed. G. S. Rousseau and P. G. Boucé (New York: Oxford University Press, 1971), 79–110.
116. Nicholas Culpeper, *The English Physician* (London: Tho. Norris, 1725), 256.
117. Freind, *Emmenologia*, 59.
118. *Aristotle's Masterpiece* (London, 1720), 25.
119. Maubray, *Female Physician*, 361.

120. See Sermon, *Ladies Companion*. On the association of the pregnant body with disease, especially in the eighteenth century, see Duden, *Woman beneath the Skin*.
121. *Aristotle's Masterpiece*, 46.
122. *Aristotle's Masterpiece*, 150–151.
123. Jean Astruc, *The Art of Midwifery Reduced to Principles* (London: J. Nourse, 1767), 150.
124. This is not to say that Smollett endorsed the virtue of physicians wholesale. In the broad satire of *Peregrine Pickle*, fraudulent and incompetent physicians are also the target of Perry's "project of revenge" (370) and Smollett's criticism. An extended analysis of Smollett's critique on the state of medicine and surgery can be read in Claude E. Jones's "Essay on the External Use of Water."
125. Lisa Cody, "The Doctor's in Labour; or, A New Whim Wham from Guildford," *Gender & History* 4 (Summer 1992): 175–196.
126. Farr, *Novel Bodies*, 123.
127. Gélis, *History of Pregnancy*, 16.
128. Gélis, *History of Pregnancy*, 142.
129. Ernelle Fife, "Gender and Professionalism in Eighteenth-Century Midwifery," *Women's Writing* 11, no. 2 (2004): 192.
130. Fife, "Gender and Professionalism," 190.
131. Fife, "Gender and Professionalism," 192.
132. Fife, "Gender and Professionalism," 198.
133. Gélis, *History of Pregnancy*, 150.
134. W. F. Bynum and Roy Porter, eds., *William Hunter and the Eighteenth-Century Medical World* (Cambridge: Cambridge University Press, 1985).
135. Lisa Forman Cody, *Birthing the Nation: Sex, Science, and the Conception of Eighteenth-Century Britons* (Oxford: Oxford University Press, 2005), 11. Male physicians often practiced midwifery even without specialization in obstetrics. See Irvine Loudon, *Medical Care and the General Practitioner, 1750–1850* (Oxford, UK: Clarendon, 1986), 86; Lord, "'Arcana of the Deity"; Josephine M. Lloyd, "The 'Languid Child' and the Eighteenth-Century Man-Midwife," *BHM* 75 (2001): 641–679.
136. Louis LaPeyre, *An Enquiry . . . Whether Women with Child Ought to Prefer the Assistance of Their Own Sex* (London: S. Blandon, 1772), 43.

## CHAPTER 4 — ROMANTIC (MIS)READINGS AND NERVOUS SYMPATHY IN CHARLOTTE LENNOX'S *THE FEMALE QUIXOTE* (1752)

1. George Cheyne, *Essay on Health and Long Life* (London: G. Strahan and J. Leake, 1724), 144.
2. Charlotte Lennox, *The Female Quixote* (Oxford: Oxford University Press, 1989), 7. Subsequent references are to this edition and are cited parenthetically in the text.
3. See Deborah Ross, "Mirror, Mirror: The Didactic Dilemma of *The Female Quixote*," *SEL* 27 (1987): 455–473; and James J. Lynch, "Romance and Realism in Charlotte Lennox's *The Female Quixote*," *Essays in Literature* 14 (1987): 51–63.
4. Margaret Anne Doody, "Shakespeare's Novels: Charlotte Lennox Illustrated," *Studies in the Novel* 19 (Fall1987): 299.
5. Laurie Langbauer, "Romance Revised: Charlotte Lennox's 'The Female Quixote,'" *NOVEL: A Forum on Fiction* 18, no. 1 (1984): 30.
6. Langbauer, "Romance Revised," 39.
7. Amelia Dale, *The Printed Reader: Gender, Quixotism, and Textual Bodies in Eighteenth-Century Britain* (Lewisburg, PA: Bucknell University Press, 2019).
8. Laurie Langbauer, *Women and Romance: The Consolations of Gender in the English Novel* (Ithaca, NY: Cornell University Press, 1990), 63.
9. Langbauer, *Women and Romance*, 85, 84.

10. Wendy Motooka, *The Age of Reasons: Quixotism, Sentimentalism, and Political Economy in Eighteenth-Century Britain* (London: Routledge, 1998), 5.
11. Susan Carlile observes that this theme of women harnessing their intelligence to protect themselves against sexual violence runs through almost all of Lennox's novels. Susan Carlile, *Charlotte Lennox: An Independent Mind* (Toronto: University of Toronto Press, 2018), 8.
12. Debra Malina, "Rereading the Patriarchal Text: *The Female Quixote, Northanger Abbey,* and the Trace of the Absent Mother," *Eighteenth-Century Fiction* 8, no. 2 (1996): 279.
13. Sara Ahmed, "A Complaint Biography," *Biography* 42, no. 3 (2019): 514–523.
14. Regina Barreca, *Untamed and Unabashed: Essays on Women and Humor in British Literature* (Detroit: Wayne State University Press, 1994), 12.
15. Audrey Bilger, *Laughing Feminism: Subversive Comedy in Frances Burney, Maria Edgeworth, and Jane Austen* (Detroit: Wayne State University Press, 1998), 9.
16. Barreca, *Untamed and Unabashed,* 30.
17. Barreca, *Untamed and Unabashed,* 45.
18. B.W. Ife, *Reading and Fiction in Golden-Age Spain: A Platonist Critique and Some Picaresque Replies* (Cambridge: Cambridge University Press, 1985), 49–83.
19. Cf. Samuel Tissot, *De la santé des gens de lettres* (1768), introduction by Francois Azouvi (Geneva: Slatkine, 1981); and Roger Chartier, "L'homme de lettres," in *L'homme des lumières,* ed. Michel Vovelle (Paris: Editions du Seuil, 1996), 159–209.
20. Thomas Laqueur, *Solitary Sex: A Cultural History of Masturbation* (New York: Zone Books, 2003).
21. Roger Chartier, *Inscription and Erasure: Literature and Written Culture from the Eleventh to the Eighteenth Century,* trans. Arthur Goldhammer (Philadelphia: University of Pennsylvania Press, 2007), 112–113.
22. Ana Vogrinçic, "The Novel-Reading Panic in 18th-Century in England: An Outline of an Early Moral Media Panic," *Medijska istraživanja* 14, no. 2 (2008): 109.
23. Charles Povey, *The Virgin in Eden; or, The State of Innocency* (London: J. Roberts, 1741), 69.
24. Thomas Trotter, *A View of the Nervous Temperament,* 3rd ed (Newcastle, UK: Walker, Longman, Hurst, Rees and Orme, 1812), 93.
25. Albrecht von Haller, *First Lines of Physiology,* vol. 1 (London: Elliot; Edinburgh: G.G.J. and J. Robinson, 1786), 218.
26. Haller, *First Lines of Physiology,* 39–40.
27. Haller, *First Lines of Physiology,* 38.
28. Haller, *First Lines of Physiology,* 34.
29. Scott Paul Gordon, "The Space of Romance in Lennox's *Female Quixote,*" *Studies in English Literature 1500–1900,* 38, no. 3 (1998): 510.
30. Carlile, *Charlotte Lennox,* 81.
31. Ildiko Csengei, *Sympathy, Sensibility and the Literature of Feeling in the Eighteenth Century* (New York: Palgrave Macmillan, 2012), 31.
32. Adam Smith, *The Theory of Moral Sentiments* (1759), ed. Knud Haakonssen (Cambridge: Cambridge University Press, 2002), 11.
33. Smith, *Theory of Moral Sentiments,* 13.
34. Christopher Lawrence, "The Nervous System and Society in the Scottish Enlightenment," in *Natural Order: Historical Studies of Scientific Culture,* ed. Barry Barnes and Steven Shapin (Beverley Hills, CA: Sage, 1979), 24–25.
35. Robert Whytt, *An Essay on the Vital and Involuntary Motions of Animals* (1751; repr., Edinburgh: John Balfour, 1763), 219–220.
36. Whytt, *Essay on the Vital and Involuntary Motions of Animals,* 270, 290, 307–316.
37. Whytt, *Essay on the Vital and Involuntary Motions of Animals,* 380.
38. Georges Canguilhem, *La formation du concept de réflexe aux XVIIe et XVIIIe siècles* (Paris: Presses Universitaires de France, 1955), 101–7.
39. Robert Whytt, *Physiological Essays* (Edinburgh: Hamilton, Balfour and Neill, 1761), 215.

40. Whytt, *Physiological Essays*, 255–256.
41. Whytt, *Essay on the Vital and Involuntary Motion of Animals*, 324–325.
42. Nima Bassiri, "The Brain and the Unconscious Soul in Eighteenth-Century Nervous Physiology: Robert Whytt's Sensorium Commune," *Journal of the History of Ideas* 74, no. 3 (2013): 425–448.
43. Whytt, *Essay on the Vital and Involuntary Motion of Animals*, 289.
44. Whytt, *Essay on the Vital and Involuntary Motion of Animals*, 310.
45. George Rousseau, "'Brainomania': Brain, Mind and Soul in the Long Eighteenth Century," *British Journal for Eighteenth-Century Studies* 30 (2007): 177.
46. Whytt, *Essay on the Vital and Involuntary Motion of Animals*, 288.
47. Francis Hutcheson, *On the Nature and Conduct of the Passions and Affections, with Illustrations on the Moral Sense* (1728), ed. Andrew Ward (Manchester, UK: Clinamen, 1999), 21, 15.
48. In Gregory Durston's examination of rape cases in eighteenth-century Britain, the most common rape victims were lower-class women, and the majority of rapists were acquaintances. Durston admits that the historical record does not necessarily reflect historical reality and suspects that most sexual assault were not reported. Gregory Durston, "Rape in the Eighteenth-Century Metropolis: Part 1," *British Journal for Eighteenth-Century Studies* 28, no. 2 (2005): 167–179; and Durston, "Rape in the Eighteenth-Century Metropolis: Part 2," *British Journal for Eighteenth-Century Studies* 29, no. 1 (2006): 15–31.
49. Motooka, *Age of Reasons*, 130.
50. Patricia Meyer Spacks, "The Subtle Sophistry of Desire: Dr. Johnson and *The Female Quixote*," *Modern Philology* 85 (1988): 532–542; Whytt, *Essay on the Vital and Involuntary Motion of Animals*, 541.
51. Ruth Perry, *Novel Relations: The Transformation of Kinship in English Literature and Culture, 1748–1818* (Cambridge: Cambridge University Press, 2004), 279.
52. Ruth Perry argues that the Hardwicke Marriage Act actually created prostitutes out of wives. Traditional sex practices before marriage were accepted before the act's passing. If single women chose the traditional route, their marriage could be rendered invalid if their marriage contracts were challenged. Perry, *Novel Relations*, 278.
53. Carlile, *Charlotte Lennox*, 8.
54. Haller, *First Lines of Physiology*, 43.
55. Stephanie Hershinow, *Born Yesterday: Inexperience and the Early Realist Novel* (Baltimore: Johns Hopkins University Press, 2020), 7.
56. Stephanie Hershinow observes that in anti-Pamelist texts like Eliza Haywood's *Anti-Pamela*, readers advocated for longer engagements in contrast to the hasty marriage exemplified in the novel, in which Pamela's virtue was questioned in her quick consent to Mr. B's proposal for marriage. Hershinow, *Born Yesterday*, 68.
57. Julia Epstein, "Marginality in Frances Burney's Novels," in *The Cambridge Companion to the English Novel*, ed. John Richetti (Cambridge: Cambridge University Press, 1996), 199.
58. Whytt, *Essay on the Vital and Involuntary Motion of Animals*, 288.
59. Eve Kosofsky Sedgwick, *Between Men: English Literature and Male Homosocial Desire* (New York: Columbia University Press, 1985), 2.
60. Lévi Strauss, *The Elementary Structures of Kinship* (Boston: Beacon, 1969), 115.
61. Heidi Hartmann, "The Unhappy Marriage of Marxism and Feminism: Towards a More Progressive Union," in *Women and Revolution: A Discussion of the Unhappy Marriage of Marxism and Feminism*, ed. Lydia Sargent (Boston: South End, 1981), 14.
62. Lynda E. Boose, "The Father's House and the Daughter in It: The Structures of Western Culture's Daughter-Father Relationship," in *Daughters and Fathers*, ed. Lynda E. Boose and Betty S. Flowers (Baltimore: Johns Hopkins University Press, 1989), 19–74.
63. Haller, *First Lines of Physiology*, 36–37.
64. Andrew Scull, *The Most Solitary of Afflictions: Madness and Society in Britain, 1700–1900* (New Haven, CT: Yale University Press, 1993), 46.
65. Scull, *Most Solitary of Afflictions*, 21.

66. For discussions of Arabella's madness, see Leland E. Warren, "Of the Conversation of Women: *The Female Quixote* and the Dream of Perfection," *Studies in Eighteenth-Century Culture* 11 (1982): 367–380; Wendy Motooka, "Coming to a Bad End: Sentimentalism, Hermeneutics, and *The Female Quixote*," *Eighteenth-Century Fiction* 8 (1996): 251–270; and Gordon, "Space of Romance," 511–512.
67. Michael McDonald, *Mystical Bedlam: Madness, Anxiety, and Healing in Seventeenth-Century England* (Cambridge: Cambridge University Press, 1981), chap. 4.
68. Warren, "Of the Conversation of Women," 370.
69. Scull, *Most Solitary of Afflictions*, 41.
70. Anna Laetitia Barbauld notes Lennox's misstep for having Arabella cured by "the Grave moralizing of a clergyman" and that she would have preferred the heroine to have "been recovered by the sense of ridicule; by falling into some absurd mistake, or by finding herself . . . the prey of some romantic footman." Barbauld would much rather Arabella learn through experience than through an infantilizing lecture. Though this chapter is titled "Being, in the Author's Opinion, the Best Chapter in this History," many regard it as an anticlimactic artistic failure. Lennox herself expressed discontentment with the novel's ending, feeling rushed to finish to earn money more quickly. Anna Laetitia Barbauld, "Mrs. Lennox," preface to *The Female Quixote*, in *The British Novelists*, vol. 24 (London: F. C. and J. Rivington, 1820). See Duncan Isles, "Johnson, Richardson, and The Female Quixote," appendix to *The Female Quixote*, ed. Margaret Dalziel (Oxford: Oxford University Press, 1970), 419–428, esp. 425–426; Carlile, *Charlotte Lennox*, 104, 109.
71. Warren, "Of the Conversation of Women," 371.
72. Catherine A. Craft, "Reworking Male Models: Aphra Behn's *Fair Vow-Breaker*, Eliza Haywood's *Fantomina*, and Charlotte Lennox's *Female Quixote*," *Modern Language Review* 86 (1991): 837.

## CODA

1. Tony McNamara, screenplay for *Poor Things*, dir. Yorgos Lanthimos (Searchlight Pictures, 2023), 94. Subsequent references are cited parenthetically in the text.
2. Fielding Blandford, *Insanity and Its Treatment* (Philadelphia: Lea, 1871), 69.
3. Marshall Hall, *Memoirs on the Nervous Systems* (London: Sherwood, Gilbert, and Piper, 1837); Johannes Müller, *Elements of Physiology* (London: Taylor and Walton, 1839–1842); Thomas Laycock, *A Treatise on the Nervous Diseases of Women* (London: Longman, Orme, Brown, Green, and Longmans, 1840); Laycock, "Reflex, Automatic, and Unconscious Cerebration: A History and Criticism," *Journal of Medical Science* 21 (1876): 1–17.
4. Andrew Scull and Diane Favreau, "The Clitoridectomy Craze," *Social Research* 53, no. 2 (1986): 245.
5. Scull and Favreau, "Clitoridectomy Craze," 247.
6. John Studd, "A Comparison of 19th Century and Current Attitudes to Female Sexuality," *Gynecological Endocrinology* 23, no. 12 (2007): 673.
7. J. M. Charcot, *Lectures on the Diseases of the Nervous System Delivered at La Salpetriere* (London, 1877).
8. Isaac Baker Brown, *On the Curability of Certain Forms of Insanity, Epilepsy, Catalepsy and Hysteria in Females* (London, 1866).
9. Charles Brown-Séquard, *Course of Lectures on the Physiology and Pathology of the Central Nervous System Delivered at the Royal College of Physicians of England in May, 1858* (Philadelphia: Collins, 1860).
10. Baker Brown, *On the Curability of Certain Forms of Insanity*, 10.
11. W. Cornish and G. Clarke, *Law and Society in England 1750–1950* (London: Sweet and Maxwell, 1989), 382–398.
12. Baker Brown, *On the Curability of Certain Forms of Insanity*, 84.
13. Barreca, *Untamed and Unabashed*, 12.

14. Schiebinger, *Mind Has No Sex?*, 191.
15. Edward Shorter, *From Paralysis to Fatigue: A History of Psychosomatic Illness in the Modern Era* (New York: Free Press, 1992).
16. T. Spencer Wells, Alfred Hegar, and Robert Battey, "Castration in Nervous Diseases: A Symposium," *American Journal of Medical Science* 92, no. 10 (1886): 442; Archibald Church, "Removal of Ovaries and Tubes in the Insane and Neurotic," *American Journal of Obstetrics and Diseases of Women and Children* 28, no. 4 (1893): 493; E. W. Cushing, "Melancholia; Masturbation; Cured by Removal of Both Ovaries," *Journal of the American Medical Association* 8 (April 1887): 442; Richard Hunter and Ida Macalpine, *Three Hundred Years of Psychiatry* (London: Oxford University Press, 1964), 861; J.E.D. Esquirol, *Mental Maladies: A Treatise on Insanity* (New York: Hafner, 1845), 339.
17. Charles D. Meigs, *Woman: Her Diseases and Remedies* (Philadelphia: Blanchard and Lea, 1848), 151; Sander Gilman, "Black Bodies, White Bodies: Toward an Iconography of Female Sexuality in Late Nineteenth-Century Art, Medicine and Literature," *Critical Inquiry* 12, no. 1 (1985): 223.
18. Baker Brown, *On the Curability of Certain Forms of Insanity*, 70. It later emerged that Baker Brown engaged in unethical behavior, operating "upon married women without the consent of their husbands, and upon unmarried women without the consent of their friends and of the patients themselves." What is more, Baker Brown threatened to commit female patients to an asylum to "frighten patients into submission, where need for operation there was none." A year after publishing his book, Baker Brown was expelled from the London Obstetric Society, and he resigned from the London Medical Society as president for failing to uphold the basis of professional honor. This was particularly sensitive for gynecologists, who "are not only the guardians of life, but, by force of circumstance, often also the guardians of female honour and purity." *British Medical Journal*, April 6, 1867, 407. For earlier examples of this accusation, see *British Medical Journal*, December 29, 1866, 729; January 12, 1867, 42; January 19, 1867, 42; January 19, 1867, 61; April 6, 1867, 388.
19. Immanuel Kant, *Kritik der Urteilskraft* (1790), in *Werke*, ed. Ernst Cassirer, vol. 5 (Berlin, 1912–1923), 199; trans. J. C. Meredith under the title *Critique of Aesthetic Judgment* (Oxford, 1911), 199–200.
20. Thomas Hobbes, *The English Works of Thomas Hobbes of Malmesbury*, ed. William Molesworth, 11 vols. (London, 1839), 4:46.
21. Aliza Rosen, "Important Abortion Cases in a Holding Pattern Following SCOTUS Decisions," Johns Hopkins: Bloomberg School of Public Health, July 3, 2024, https://publichealth.jhu.edu/2024/scotus-mifepristone-and-emtala-decisions-explained#:~:text=For%20now%2C%20mifepristone%20remains%20on,fire%20again%20in%20the%20future.
22. Amy Howe, "Supreme Court Appears Likely to Allow Abortion Drug to Remain Available," *Scotusblog*, March 26, 2024, https://www.scotusblog.com/2024/03/supreme-court-appears-likely-to-allow-abortion-drug-to-remain-available/.
23. Rosen, "Important Abortion Cases."

# BIBLIOGRAPHY


Ackermann, Jacob. *Über den Einfluss des Geschlechts-Unterschiedes auf Ausbildung und Heilung von Krankheiten*. Stendal, 1829.

Adelman, Janet. "Making Defect Perfection: Shakespeare and the One-Sex Model." In *Enacting Gender on the Renaissance Stage*, edited by Viviana Comensoli and Anne Russell, 23–52. Urbana: University of Illinois Press, 1999.

Ahern, Stephen. *Affected Sensibilities: Romantic Excess and the Genealogy of the Novel*. New York: AMS Press, 2007.

———. "Nothing More than Feelings? Affect Theory Reads the Age of Sensibility." *Eighteenth Century: Theory and Interpretation* 58, no. 3 (2017): 281–295.

Ahmed, Sara. "A Complaint Biography." *Biography* 42, no. 3 (2019): 514–523.

Allen, Peter Lewis. *The Wages of Sin: Sex and Disease, Past and Present*. Chicago: University of Chicago Press, 2000.

Allestree, Richard. *The Ladies Calling*. 5th ed. Oxford, UK, 1677.

Alter, Robert. *Fielding and the Nature of the Novel*. Cambridge, MA: Harvard University Press, 1968.

*Arbor Vitae; or, The Natural History of the Tree of Life*. London: E. Hill, 1741.

Aristotle. *Generation of Animals*. Translated by A. Platt. In *The Complete Works of Aristotle*. Edited by J. Barnes. Princeton, NJ: Princeton University Press, 1984.

*Aristotle's Masterpiece*. London, 1720.

Armstrong, John. *The Oeconomy of Love: A Poetical Essay*. London: T. Cooper, 1736.

Armstrong, Nancy. *Desire and Domestic Fiction: A Political History of the Novel*. New York: Oxford University Press, 1987.

Arnaud, Sabine. *On Hysteria: The Invention of a Medical Category between 1670 and 1820*. Chicago: University of Chicago Press, 2015.

Astruc, Jean. *The Art of Midwifery Reduced to Principles*. London: J. Nourse, 1767.

———. *A Treatise on All the Diseases Incident to Women Containing an Account of Their Causes, Differences, Symptoms, Diagnostics, Prognostics and Cure, Translated from a Manuscript of the Author's Lectures Read at Paris, 1740*. London: M. Cooper, 1743.

Austin, Andrea. "Shooting Blanks: Potency, Parody, and Eliza Haywood's *The History of Miss Betsy Thoughtless*." In *The Passionate Fictions of Eliza Haywood*, edited by Kirsten T. Saxton and Rebecca P. Bocchicchio, 259–282. Lexington: University Press of Kentucky, 2000.

Baines, Paul. "Joseph Andrews." In *The Cambridge Companion to Henry Fielding*, edited by Claude Rawson, 50–64. Cambridge: Cambridge University Press, 2007.

Baker Brown, Isaac. *On the Curability of Certain Forms of Insanity, Epilepsy, Catalepsy and Hysteria in Females*. London, 1866.

Bakhtin, Mikhail. *The Dialogic Imagination: Four Essays*. Edited by Michael Holquist. Translated by Caryl Emerson and Michael Holquist. Austin: University of Texas Press, 1981.

———. *Rabelais and His World*. Translated by Hélène Iswolsky. Bloomington: Indiana University Press, 1984.

Ball, John. *The Female Physician; or, Every Woman Her Own Doctor*. London, 1777.

Ballaster, Ros. *Seductive Forms: Women's Amatory Fiction from 1684 to 1740*. Oxford: Oxford University Press, 1992.

Barbauld, Anna Laetitia. Preface to *The Female Quixote*. In *The British Novelists*, vol. 24, i–iv. London: F. C. and J. Rivington, 1820.

Barreca, Regina. *Untamed and Unabashed: Essays on Women and Humor in British Literature*. Detroit: Wayne State University Press, 1994.

Bassiri, Nima. "The Brain and the Unconscious Soul in Eighteenth-Century Nervous Physiology: Robert Whytt's Sensorium Commune." *Journal of the History of Ideas* 74, no. 3 (2013): 425–448.

Battestin, Martin C. *The Moral Basis of Fielding's Art: A Study of "Joseph Andrews."* Middletown, CT: Wesleyan University Press, 1959.

Beasley, Jerry. *Tobias Smollett: Novelist*. Athens: University of Georgia Press, 1998.

Beattie, James. "Essay on Laughter and Ludicrous Composition." In *Essays*, 3rd ed., 321–486. London: Edward and Charles Dilly, 1779.

*Beauty's Triumph, or, the Superiority of the Fair Sex Invariably Proved*. London: J. Robinson, 1751.

Bender, John. *Ends of Enlightenment*. Stanford, CA: Stanford University Press, 2012.

Berlant, Lauren, and Sianne Ngai. "Comedy Has Issues." *Critical Inquiry* 43, no. 2 (2017): 233–249.

Berlant, Lauren, and Michael Warner. "Sex in Public." *Critical Inquiry* 24 (1998): 548–566.

Bilger, Audrey. *Laughing Feminism: Subversive Comedy in Frances Burney, Maria Edgeworth, and Jane Austen*. Detroit: Wayne State University Press, 1998.

Biology and Gender Study Group. "The Importance of Feminist Critique for Contemporary Cell Biology." In *Feminism and Science*, edited by Nancy Tuana, 172–187. Bloomington: Indiana University Press, 1989.

Birke, Lynda. *Feminism and the Biological Body*. New Brunswick, NJ: Rutgers University Press, 2000.

———. *Women, Feminism and Biology: The Feminist Challenge*. New York: Methuen, 1986.

Blackmore, Richard. "An Essay upon Wit." In *Essays upon Several Subjects*, 190–230. 1716. Reprint, New York: Garland, 1971.

———. *A Treatise of the Spleen and Vapours; or Hypochondriacal and Hysterical Affections. With Three Discourses on the Nature and Cure of the Cholick, Melancholy, and Palsies*. London: Pemberton, 1726.

Blandford, Fielding. *Insanity and Its Treatment*. Philadelphia: Lea, 1871.

Blondel, James Augustus. *The Strength of Imagination in Pregnant Women*. London: J. Peele, 1727.

Boerhaave, Herman. *Boerhaave's Aphorisms: Concerning the Knowledge and Cure of Diseases*. London: W. Innys and C. Hitch, 1728.

Boose, Lynda E. "The Father's House and the Daughter in It: The Structures of Western Culture's Daughter-Father Relationship." In *Daughters and Fathers*, edited by Lynda E. Boose and Betty S. Flowers, 19–74. Baltimore: Johns Hopkins University Press, 1989.

Boswell, James. *Life of Johnson*. Edited by George B. Hill. 4 vols. Oxford: Oxford University Press, 1994.

Boucé, Paul-Gabriel. "Imagination, Pregnant Women, and Monsters, in Eighteenth-Century England and France." In *Sexual Underworlds of the Enlightenment*, edited by G. S. Rousseau and Roy Porter, 86–100. Chapel Hill: University of North Carolina Press, 1988.

Bowen, Scarlet. "'A Sawce-box and Boldface Indeed': Refiguring the Female Servant in the Pamela-Antipamela Debate." *Studies in Eighteenth-Century Culture* 28 (1999): 257–285.

Bowers, Toni. "'A Point of Conscience': Breastfeeding and Maternal Authority in *Pamela*, Part 2." In *Inventing Maternity: Politics, Science, and Literature, 1650–1865*, edited by Susan C. Greenfield and Carol Barash, 138–158. Lexington: University Press of Kentucky, 1999.

Breitenberg, Mark. *Anxious Masculinity in Early Modern England*. Cambridge: Cambridge University Press, 1996.

Brewer, John. *The Pleasures of the Imagination: English Culture in the Eighteenth Century*. New York: Farrar, Straus and Giroux, 1997.

Broomhall, Susan, ed. *Spaces for Feeling: Gender, Affect, and Sociability in Britain, 1650–1850.* New York: Routledge, 2015.

Brown-Séquard, Charles. *Course of Lectures on the Physiology and Pathology of the Central Nervous System Delivered at the Royal College of Physicians of England in May, 1858.* Philadelphia: Collins, 1860.

Buchan, William. *Domestic Medicin[e]; or, The Family Physician.* London: John Dunlap, 1772.

Buckley, Jennifer. *Gender, Pregnancy and Power in Eighteenth-Century Literature: The Maternal Imagination.* Cham, Switzerland: Palgrave Macmillan, 2017.

Bynum, W. F., and Roy Porter, eds. *William Hunter and the Eighteenth-Century Medical World.* Cambridge: Cambridge University Press, 1985.

Canguilhem, Georges. *La formation du concept de réflexe aux XVIIe et XVIIIe siècles.* Paris: Presses Universitaires de France, 1955.

Carlile, Susan. *Charlotte Lennox: An Independent Mind.* Toronto: University of Toronto Press, 2018.

Carter, Elizabeth. *Letters from Mrs. Elizabeth Carter to Mrs. Montagu, 1755–1800.* Edited by Montagu Pennington. London: F. C and J. Rivington,1817.

Castle, Terry. *Clarissa's Cyphers: Meaning and Disruption in Richardson's "Clarissa."* Ithaca, NY: Cornell University Press, 1982.

———. *Masquerades and Civilization: The Carnivalesque in Eighteenth-Century Culture and Fiction.* Stanford, CA: Stanford University Press, 1986.

[Chapone, Sarah]. *The Hardship of the English Laws in Relation to Wives.* London: W. Boyer, 1735.

Charcot, J. M. *Lectures on the Diseases of the Nervous System Delivered at La Salpetriere.* London, 1877.

Chartier, Roger. *Inscription and Erasure: Literature and Written Culture from the Eleventh to the Eighteenth Century.* Translated by Arthur Goldhammer. Philadelphia: University of Pennsylvania Press, 2007.

———. "L'homme de lettres." In *L'homme des lumières*, edited by Michel Vovelle, 159–209. Paris: Editions du Seuil, 1996.

Cheyne, George. *Essay on Health and Long Life.* London: G. Strahan and J. Leake, 1724.

Chico, Tita. *The Experimental Imagination: Literary Knowledge and Science in the British Enlightenment.* Stanford, CA: Stanford University Press, 2018.

Chow, Jeremy. "Mare Mortis: Blackness, Ecology, & 'Kinlessness' in Neville's *The Isle of Pines.*" *Atlantic Studies* 18, no. 2 (2021): 1–17.

Church, Archibald. "Removal of Ovaries and Tubes in the Insane and Neurotic." *American Journal of Obstetrics and Diseases of Women and Children* 28, no. 4 (1893): 491–498.

Cody, Lisa Forman. *Birthing the Nation: Sex, Science, and the Conception of Eighteenth-Century Britons.* Oxford: Oxford University Press, 2005.

———. "The Doctor's in Labour; or, A New Whim Wham from Guildford." *Gender & History* 4 (Summer 1992): 175–196.

Cohen, Ted. *Jokes: Philosophical Thoughts on Joking Matters.* Chicago: University of Chicago Press, 1999.

Colburn, Glen. "Struggling Manfully through Henry Fielding's *Amelia*: Hysteria, Medicine, and the Novel in Eighteenth-Century England." *Studies in Eighteenth-Century Culture* 26 (1997): 87–123.

Collins, R. G. "The Hidden Bastard: A Question of Illegitimacy in Smollett's *Peregrine Pickle.*" *PMLA* 94, no. 1 (1979): 91–105.

Cook, Elizabeth Heckendorn. *Epistolary Bodies: Gender and Genre in the Eighteenth-Century Republic of Letters.* Stanford, CA: Stanford University Press, 1996.

Cooper, Anthony Ashley, Third Earl of Shaftesbury. *Characteristics of Men, Manners, Opinions, Times with a Collection of Letters by the Right Honorable* ***Anthony*** *Shaftesbury.* Vol. 3. Basil: Tourneisen and Legrand, 1790.

Cornish, W., and G. Clarke. *Law and Society in England 1750–1950.* London: Sweet and Maxwell, 1989.

Craft, Catherine A. "Reworking Male Models: Aphra Behn's *Fair Vow-Breaker*, Eliza Haywood's *Fantomina*, and Charlotte Lennox's *Female Quixote*." *Modern Language Review* 86 (1991): 821–838.

Crawford, Katherine B. *Eunuchs and Castrati: Disability and Normativity in Early Modern Europe.* London: Routledge, 2018.

Crawford, Patricia. "Women's Published Writings 1600–1700." In *Women in English Society 1500–1800*, edited by Mary Prior, 211–282. London: Methuen, 1985.

Csengei, Ildiko. *Sympathy, Sensibility and the Literature of Feeling in the Eighteenth Century.* New York: Palgrave Macmillan, 2012.

Cullen, William. *First Lines of the Practice of Physic.* Vol. 2. Edinburgh: Reid and Bathgate, 1784.

Culpeper, Nicholas. *A Directory for Midwives.* London: J. and A. Churchill, 1701.

———. *The English Physician.* London: Tho. Norris, 1725.

Cushing, E. W. "Melancholia; Masturbation; Cured by Removal of Both Ovaries." *Journal of the American Medical Association* 8 (April 1887): 441–442.

Dale, Amelia. *The Printed Reader: Gender, Quixotism, and Textual Bodies in Eighteenth-Century Britain.* Lewisburg, PA: Bucknell University Press, 2019.

Darwin, Erasmus. *Zoomonia; or, The Laws of Organic Life.* London: J. Johnson, 1794.

Davis, Lennerd J. *Bending Over Backwards: Disability, Dismodernism, and Other Difficult Positions.* New York: New York University Press, 2002.

———. "Dr. Johnson, Amelia, and the Discourse of Disability in the Eighteenth Century." In *"Defects": Engendering the Modern Body*, edited by Helen Deutsch and Felicity Nussbaum, 54–74. Ann Arbor: University of Michigan Press, 2000.

Dean-Jones, Lesley-Ann. *Women's Bodies in Classical Greek Science.* Oxford, UK: Clarendon, 1996.

Defoe, Daniel. *Compleat English Gentleman.* Edited by Karl D. Bülbring. Edinburgh: Ballantyne, 2006.

———. *Conjugal Lewdness; or, Matrimonial Whoredom. A Treatise concerning the Use and Abuse of the Marriage Bed.* 1727. Reprint, Gainesville, FL: Scholars' Facsimiles and Reprints, 1967.

Deleurye, F. A. "Des passions de l'ame." In *Traité des accouchemens en faveur des élèves.* Paris, 1770.

Deutsch, Helen, and Felicity Nussbaum. Introduction to *"Defects": Engendering the Modern Body*, edited by Helen Deutsch and Felicity Nussbaum, 1–28. Ann Arbor: University of Michigan Press, 2000.

Dickie, Simon. *Cruelty and Laughter: Forgotten Comic Literature and the Unsentimental Eighteenth Century.* Chicago: University of Chicago Press, 2011.

———. "Hilarity and Pitilessness in the Mid-Eighteenth Century: English Jestbook Humor." *Eighteenth-Century Studies* 37, no. 1 (2003): 1–22.

———. "Tobias Smollett and the Ramble Novel." In *The Oxford History of the Novel in English*, vol. 2, *English and British Fiction, 1750–1820*, edited by Peter Garside and Karen O'Brien, 92–108. New York: Oxford University Press, 2015.

Dixon, Thomas. *From Passions to Emotions: The Creation of a Secular Psychological Category.* Cambridge: Cambridge University Press, 2003.

Dobson, Austin. *Eighteenth-Century Vignettes: Second Series.* London: Chatto and Windus, 1894.

Donahue, Frank. "Colonizing Readers: Review Criticism and the Formation of a Reading Public." In *The Consumption of Culture: Image, Object, Text*, edited by Ann Bermingham and John Brewer, 57–74. London: Routledge, 1995.

Donne, John. *The Complete English Poems.* London: Penguin, 2004. Ebook.

Donoghue, Emma. *Passions between Women: British Lesbian Culture 1668–1801.* New York: Harper Perennial, 1996.

Doody, Margaret Anne. "Shakespeare's Novels: Charlotte Lennox Illustrated." *Studies in the Novel* 19 (Fall 1987): 296–310.

Douglas, Aileen. *Uneasy Sensations: Smollett and the Body*. Chicago: University of Chicago Press, 1994.

Dryden, John. *A Discourse Concerning the Original and Progress of Satire*. In *The Satires of Decimus Junius Juvenalis: Translated into English Verse by Mr. Dryden and Several Other Eminent Hands*, i–xxxix. London: Jacob Tonson, 1693.

———. *An Evening's Love or the Mockastrologer*. In *The Works of John Dryden*, vol. 10, edited by Maximillian G. Novak and George R. Guffey, 195–314. Berkeley: University of California Press, 1970.

Duden, Barbara. *The Woman beneath the Skin: A Doctor's Patients in Seventeenth-Century Germany*. Cambridge: Cambridge University Press, 1991.

Dulaure, Jacques-Antoine. *Pogonologia; or A Philosophical and Historical Essay on Beards. Translated from the French*. Exeter, 1786.

D'Urfey, Thomas. *Scandalum magnatum, or, Potapski's Case, A Satyr against Polish Oppression*. London, 1682.

Durston, Gregory. "Rape in the Eighteenth-Century Metropolis: Part 1." *British Journal for Eighteenth-Century Studies* 28, no. 2 (2005): 167–179.

———. "Rape in the Eighteenth-Century Metropolis: Part 2." *British Journal for Eighteenth-Century Studies* 29, no. 1 (2006): 15–31.

Ehlers, Leigh A. "Mrs. Shandy's 'Lint and Basilicon': The Importance of Women in *Tristram Shandy*." *South Atlantic Review* 46 (1981): 61–73.

Empson, William. "Tom Jones." *Kenyon Review* 20 (1958): 217–259. Reprinted in *Fielding: A Collection of Critical Essays*, edited by Ronald Paulson, 124–126. Englewood Cliffs, NJ: Prentice Hall, 1962.

Epstein, Julia. "Marginality in Frances Burney's Novels." In *The Cambridge Companion to the English Novel*, edited by John Richetti, 198–211. Cambridge: Cambridge University Press, 1996.

———. "The Pregnant Imagination, Women's Bodies, and Fetal Rights." In *Inventing Maternity: Politics, Science, and Literature, 1650–1865*, edited by Susan C. Greenfield and Carol Barash, 111–137. Lexington: University Press of Kentucky, 1999.

Esquirol, J.E.D. *Mental Maladies: A Treatise on Insanity*. New York: Hafner, 1845.

Exton, Brudenell. *A New and General System of Midwifery in Four Parts*. London: W. Owen, 1753.

Fairchilds, Cissie. *Domestic Enemies: Servants and Their Masters in Old Regime France*. Baltimore: Johns Hopkins University Press, 2019.

Farr, Jason. *Novel Bodies: Disability and Sexuality in Eighteenth-Century British Literature*. Lewisburg, PA: Bucknell University Press, 2019.

Faurot, Ruth. "Mrs. Shandy Observed." *Studies in English Literature* 10 (1970): 579–589.

Fergus, Jan. "Provincial Servants' Reading in the Late Eighteenth Century." In *The Practice and Representation of Reading in England*, edited by Helen Small and Naomi Tadmor, 202–225. Cambridge: Cambridge University Press, 1996.

Fielding, Henry. *An Apology for the Life of Mrs. Shamela Andrews*. 1741. Edited by Douglas Brooks-Davies. Oxford: Oxford University Press, 1999.

———. *Joseph Andrews*. 1741. Edited by Douglas Brooks-Davies. Oxford: Oxford University Press, 1999.

———. *"Joseph Andrews" and "Shamela."* Edited by Martin C. Battestin. Boston: Houghton Mifflin, 1961.

———. *Tom Jones*. 1749. Edited by John Bender and Simon Stern. Oxford: Oxford University Press, 1996.

Fielding, Henry, and Sarah Fielding. *Correspondence of Henry and Sarah Fielding*. Edited by Martin C. Battestin and Clive T. Probyn. Oxford, UK: Clarendon, 1993.

Fife, Ernelle. "Gender and Professionalism in Eighteenth-Century Midwifery." *Women's Writing* 11, no. 2 (2004): 185–200.

Filmer, Robert. *Patriarcha and Other Writings*. Edited by Johann P. Sommerville. Cambridge: Cambridge University Press, 1991.

Fish, Stanley. *Is There a Text in This Class? The Authority of Interpretive Communities*. Cambridge, MA: Harvard University Press, 1980.

Fissell, Mary Elizabeth. *Vernacular Bodies: The Politics of Reproduction in Early Modern England*. Oxford: Oxford University Press, 2004.

Foucault, Michel. *The History of Sexuality*. Vol. 1, *An Introduction*. New York: Pantheon Books, 1978.

———. *Madness and Civilization: A History of Insanity in the Age of Reason*. New York: Pantheon Books, 1961.

Fox, Adam. "Popular Verses and Their Readership in the Early Seventeenth Century." In *The Practice and Representation of Reading in England*, edited by James Raven, Helen Small, and Naomi Tadmor, 125–137. Cambridge: Cambridge University Press, 1996.

Francus, Marilyn. "The Monstrous Mother: Reproductive Anxiety in Swift and Pope." *ELH* 61, no. 4 (1994): 829–851.

Frank, Judith. *Common Ground: Eighteenth-Century English Satiric Fiction and the Poor*. Stanford, CA: Stanford University Press, 1997.

Freind, John. *Emmenologia*. Translated by Thomas Dale. London: T. Cox, 1729.

Freud, Sigmund. *Jokes and Their Relation to the Unconscious*. London: Penguin, 2002.

Frye, Northrop. *Anatomy of Criticism: Four Essays*. Princeton, NJ: Princeton University Press, 1957.

Ftacek, Julia. "Jonathan Swift and the Transgender Classroom." *Journal for Eighteenth-Century Studies* 43, no. 3 (2020): 303–314.

Gallagher, Catherine. *Nobody's Story: The Vanishing Acts of Women Writers in the Marketplace, 1670–1820*. Berkeley: University of California Press, 1994.

Gaub, Jerome. *De regimine mentis*. 1747. Translated by L. J. Rather. Berkeley: University of California Press, 1965.

Gautier, Gary. "Marriage and Family in Fielding's Fiction." *Studies in the Novel* 27, no. 2 (1995): 111–128.

Gélis, Jacques. *History of Childbirth: Fertility, Pregnancy, and Birth in Early Modern Europe*. Boston: Northeastern University Press, 1991.

Gilman, Sander. "Black Bodies, White Bodies: Toward an Iconography of Female Sexuality in Late Nineteenth-Century Art, Medicine and Literature." *Critical Inquiry* 12, no. 1 (1985): 204–242.

Gordon, Scott Paul. "The Space of Romance in Lennox's Female Quixote." *Studies in English Literature 1500–1900*, 38, no. 3 (1998): 499–516.

Gowing, Laura. *Common Bodies: Women, Touch, and Power in Seventeenth-Century England*. New Haven, CT: Yale University Press, 2003.

Greenfield, Susan C. "Aborting the 'Mother Plot': Politics and Generation in *Absolom and Achitophel*." In *Inventing Maternity: Politics, Science, and Literature, 1650–1865*, edited by Susan C. Greenfield and Carol Barash, 86–110. Lexington: University Press of Kentucky, 1999.

Grigg, John. *Advice to the Female Sex in General, Particularly Those in a State of Pregnancy and Lying-In: The Complaints Incident to Their Respective Situations Are Specified, and Treatment Recommended, Agreeable to Modern Practice*. Bath, UK: S. Hazard, 1789.

Grosz, Elizabeth. *Volatile Bodies: Toward a Corporeal Feminism*. Bloomington: Indiana University Press, 1994.

Gubar, Susan. "The Female Monster in Augustan Satire." *Signs* 3 (1977): 380–394.

Guillén, Claudio. *Literature as System: Essays toward the Theory of Literary History*. Princeton, NJ: Princeton University Press, 2015.

Halberstam, Jack. *Female Masculinity*. Durham, NC: Duke University Press, 2018.

Hall, Marshall. *Memoirs on the Nervous Systems*. London: Sherwood, Gilbert, and Piper, 1837.

Haller, Albrecht von. *First Lines of Physiology*. Vol. 1. London: Elliot; Edinburgh: G. G. J. and J. Robinson, 1786.
Hamilton, Alexander. *A Treatise of Midwifery Comprehending the Management of Female Complaints, and the Treatment of Children in Early Infancy—Divested of Technical Terms and Abstruse Theories*. London: J. Murray; Edinburgh: Dickson, Creech, and Elliot, 1781.
Hare, Edward. "The History of 'Nervous Disorders' from 1600 to 1840, and a Comparison with Modern Views." *British Journal of Psychiatry* 159, no. 1 (1991): 37–45.
Harley, David. "Provincial Midwives in England: Lancashire and Cheshire, 1660–1760." In *The Art of Midwifery: Early Modern Midwives in Europe*, edited by Hilary Marland, 27–58. London: Routledge, 1993.
Harris, Jocelyn. *Samuel Richardson*. Cambridge: Cambridge University Press, 1987.
Harrow, Sharon. "Having Text: Desire and Language in Haywood's *Love in Excess* and *The Distressed Orphan*." *Eighteenth Century Fiction* 22, no. 2 (2009): 279–308.
Hartmann, Heidi. "The Unhappy Marriage of Marxism and Feminism: Towards a More Progressive Union." In *Women and Revolution: A Discussion of the Unhappy Marriage of Marxism and Feminism*, edited by Lydia Sargent, 1–41. Boston: South End, 1981.
Harvey, Karen. "Epochs of Embodiment: Men, Women and the Material Body." *Journal for Eighteenth-Century Studies* 42, no. 4 (2019): 455–469.
Harvey, William. *Anatomic Exercises on the Generation of Animals*. In *The Works of William Harvey*, translated by Robert Willis, 145–588. London: Sydenham Society, 1847.
Hawley, Judith. "The Anatomy of *Tristram Shandy*." *Literature and Medicine during the Eighteenth Century*. London: Routledge, 1993: 84–100.
Haywood, Eliza. *Fantomina and Other Works*. Edited by Alexander Pettit, Margaret Case Croskery, and Anna C. Patchias. Peterborough, ON: Broadview, 2004.
———. *The Female Spectator*. 1744–1746. In *Selected Works of Eliza Haywood*, edited by Kathryn R. King and Alexander Pettit, vols. 1–2. London: Pickering and Chatto, 2001.
———. *The Injur'd Husband; or, The Mistaken Resentment and Lasselia; or, The Self-Abandon'd*. 1722. Edited by Jerry C. Beasley. Lexington: University Press of Kentucky, 1999.
———. *Love in Excess; or, The Fatal Enquiry*. 1719. Edited by David Oakleaf. Peterborough, ON: Broadview, 2000.
Haywood, Eliza Fowler. *Life's Progress through the Passions: or, the Adventures of Natura*. London: T. Gardner, 1748.
Hazlitt, William. "Lecture I—Introductory: On Wit and Humour." In *Lectures on the Comic Writers, Etc. of Great Britain*, edited by A. R. Waller and Arnold Glover. London: J. M. Dent, 1903.
Hershinow, Stephanie. *Born Yesterday: Inexperience and the Early Realist Novel*. Baltimore: Johns Hopkins University Press, 2020.
[Hewardine, William?]. *Hilaria, the Festive Board*. Printed for the Author, 1798.
Highmore, Nathaniel. *The History of Generation*. London: John Martin, 1651.
Hirschman, A. O. *The Passions and the Interests*. Princeton, NJ: Princeton University Press, 1977.
Hobbes, Thomas. *De Cive: The English Version*. 1642. Edited by Howard Warrender. Oxford, UK: Clarendon, 1983.
———. *The English Works of Thomas Hobbes of Malmesbury*. Edited by William Molesworth. 11 vols. London: Bohn, 1839.
———. *Leviathan*. 1651. Edited by C. B. Macpherson. Harmondsworth, UK: Penguin, 1985.
Hopkins, Lisa. "Marriage as Comic Closure." In *The Shakespearean Marriage*, 16–33. London: Palgrave Macmillan, 1998.
Howe, Amy. "Supreme Court Appears Likely to Allow Abortion Drug to Remain Available." *Scotusblog*, March 26, 2024. https://www.scotusblog.com/2024/03/supreme-court-appears-likely-to-allow-abortion-drug-to-remain-available/.
Huet, Marie-Hélène. *Monstrous Imagination*. Cambridge, MA: Harvard University Press, 1993.
Hultquist, Aleksondra. "Eliza Haywood's Progress through the Passions." In *Passions, Sympathy and Print Culture: Public Opinion and Emotional Authenticity in Eighteenth-Century Britain*,

edited by Heather Kerr, David Lemmings, and Robert Phiddian, 86–104. New York: Palgrave Macmillan, 2016.

Hunter, J. Paul. *Before Novels: The Cultural Contexts of Eighteenth-Century English Fiction*. New York: Norton, 1990.

Hunter, Richard, and Ida Macalpine. *Three Hundred Years of Psychiatry*. London: Oxford University Press, 1964.

Hutcheson, Francis. *On the Nature and Conduct of the Passions and Affections, with Illustrations on the Moral Sense*. 1728. Edited by Andrew Ward. Manchester, UK: Clinamen, 1999.

———. *Reflections upon Laughter, and Remarks on the Fable of the Bees*. Glasgow: R. Urie, 1750.

Ife, B. W. *Reading and Fiction in Golden-Age Spain: A Platonist Critique and Some Picaresque Replies*. Cambridge: Cambridge University Press, 1985.

Ingrassia, Catherine. Introduction to *Anti-Pamela and Shamela*, edited by Catherine Ingrassia, 7–43. Peterborough, ON: Broadview, 2004.

Irigaray, Luce. "This Sex Which Is Not One." In *This Sex Which Is Not One*, 23–33. Ithaca, NY: Cornell University Press, 1985.

Isles, Duncan. "Johnson, Richardson, and *The Female Quixote*." Appendix to *The Female Quixote*, edited by Margaret Dalziel, 419–428. Oxford: Oxford University Press, 1970.

Jackson, Kate. *George Newnes and the New Journalism in Britain 1880–1910: Culture and Profit*. Aldershot, UK: Ashgate, 2001.

Johnstone, W. *William Smellie: The Master of British Midwifery*. Edinburgh: E & S Livingstone, 1952.

Jones, Claude E. "An Essay on the External Use of Water, by Tobias Smollett." *Bulletin of the Institute of the History of Medicine* 3, no. 1 (1935): 31–82.

Jordanova, Ludmilla. "Gender, Generation, and Science: William Hunter's Obstetrical Atlas." In *William Hunter and the Eighteenth-Century Medical World*, edited by W. F. Bynum and Roy Porter, 402–412. Cambridge: Cambridge University Press, 1985.

———. "Interrogating the Concept of Reproduction in the Eighteenth Century." In *Conceiving the New World Order: The Global Politics of Reproduction*, edited by Faye Ginsburg and Rayna Rapp, 369–386. Berkeley: University of California Press, 1995.

———. *Sexual Visions: Images of Gender in Science and Medicine between the Eighteenth and Twentieth Centuries*. Madison: University of Wisconsin Press, 1989.

Joshua, Essaka. "Disability and Deformity: Function Impairment and Aesthetics in the Long Eighteenth Century." In *The Cambridge Companion to Literature and Disability*, edited by Clare Barker and Stuart Murray, 47–61. Cambridge: Cambridge University Press, 2018.

Kant, Immanuel. *Beobachtungen uber das Gefuhl des Schonen und Erhabenen*. In *Kants Werke*, edited by Wilhelm Dilthey, 207–256. Berlin, 1900–1919.

———. *Critique of Judgement*. Translated by James Creed Meredith and Nicholas Walker. Oxford: Oxford University Press, 2007.

———. *Kritik der Urteilskraft*. 1790. In *Werke*, edited by Ernst Cassirer, vol. 5, 199. Berlin, 1912–1923. Translated by J. C. Meredith under the title *Critique of Aesthetic Judgment*. Oxford, UK, 1911.

Kaplan, E. Ann. *Motherhood and Representation: The Mother in Popular Culture and Melodrama*. London: Routledge, 1992.

Keeling, Kara. *Queer Times, Black Futures*. New York: New York University Press, 2019.

Keiser, Jess. *Nervous Fictions: Literary Form and the Enlightenment Origins of Neuroscience*. Charlottesville: University of Virginia Press, 2020.

Kelleher, Paul. *Making Love: Sentiment and Sexuality in Eighteenth-Century British Literature*. Lewisburg, PA: Bucknell University Press, 2015.

Keller, Eve. "Embryonic Individuals: The Rhetoric of Seventeenth-Century Embryology and the Construction of Early-Modern Identity." *Eighteenth-Century Studies* 33, no. 3 (2000): 321–348.

———. "Making Up for Losses: The Workings of Gender in William Harvey's *de Generatione animalium*." In *Inventing Maternity: Politics, Science, and Literature, 1650–1865*, edited by

Susan C. Greenfield and Carol Barash, 34–56. Lexington: University Press of Kentucky, 1999.

Keller, Evelyn Fox. *Reflections on Gender and Science*. New Haven, CT: Yale University Press, 1985.

Kerr, Heather, David Lemmings, and Robert Phiddian, eds. *Passions, Sympathy and Print Culture: Public Opinion and Emotional Authenticity in Eighteenth-Century Britain*. New York: Palgrave Macmillan, 2016.

Keymer, Thomas. Introduction to *"Joseph Andrews" and "Shamela,"* edited by Douglas Brooks-Davies, ix–xxxv. Oxford: Oxford University Press, 1999.

Keymer, Thomas, and Peter Sabor, eds. *The Pamela Controversy: Criticisms and Adaptations of Samuel Richardson's "Pamela," 1740–1750*. 6 vols. London: Pickering and Chatto, 2001.

King, Helen. *The One-Sex Body on Trial: The Classical and Early Modern Evidence*. Burlington, VT: Ashgate, 2013.

King, Kathryn R. "Henry and Eliza: Feudlings or Friends?" In *Henry Fielding in Our Time: Papers Presented at the Tercentenary Conference*, edited by J. A. Downie, 215–231. Newcastle upon Tyne, UK: Cambridge Scholars, 2008.

King, Lester S. *The Medical World of the Eighteenth Century*. Chicago: University of Chicago Press, 1958.

Klein, Ula Lukszo. "Eighteenth-Century Female Cross-Dressers and Their Beards." *Journal for Early Modern Cultural Studies* 16, no. 4 (2016): 119–143.

Koch-Rein, Anson. "*Trans*-lating the Monster: Transgender Affect and *Frankenstein*." *LIT: Literature Interpretation Theory* 30, no. 1 (2019): 44–61.

Langbauer, Laurie. "Romance Revised: Charlotte Lennox's 'The Female Quixote.'" *NOVEL: A Forum on Fiction* 18, no. 1 (1984): 29–49.

———. *Women and Romance: The Consolations of Gender in the English Novel*. Ithaca, NY: Cornell University Press, 1990.

Lanser, Susan S. "Novel (Lesbian) Subjects: The Sexual History of Form." *Novel: A Forum on Fiction* 42 (2009): 497–503.

———. "Sapphic Dialogics: Historical Narratology and the Sexuality of Form." In *Postclassical Narratology: New Essays*, edited by Monika Fludernik and Jan Alber, 186–205. Columbus: Ohio State University Press, 2010.

LaPeyre, Louis. *An Enquiry . . . Whether Women with Child Ought to Prefer the Assistance of Their Own Sex*. London: S. Blandon, 1772.

Laqueur, Thomas. *Making Sex: Body and Gender from the Greeks to Freud*. Cambridge, MA: Harvard University Press, 1992.

———. "Orgasm, Generation, and the Politics of Reproductive Biology." In *The Making of the Modern Body: Sexuality and Society in the Nineteenth Century*, edited by Catherine Gallagher and Thomas Laqueur, 1–41. Berkeley: University of California Press, 1987.

———. *Solitary Sex: A Cultural History of Masturbation*. New York: Zone Books, 2003.

Larner, Christina. *Enemies of God: The Witch-Hunt in Scotland*. Baltimore: Johns Hopkins University Press, 1981.

Lau, Travis Chi Wing. "Defoe before Immunity: A Prophylactic *Journal of the Plague Year*." *Digital Defoe* 11 (2019): 23–39.

Lawrence, Christopher. "The Nervous System and Society in the Scottish Enlightenment." In *Natural Order: Historical Studies of Scientific Culture*, edited by Barry Barnes and Steven Shapin, 24–25. Beverley Hills, CA: Sage, 1979.

Laycock, Thomas. "Reflex, Automatic, and Unconscious Cerebration: A History and Criticism." *Journal of Medical Science* 21 (1876): 1–17.

———. *A Treatise on the Nervous Diseases of Women*. London: Longman, Orme, Brown, Green, and Longmans, 1840.

Leake, John. *Medical instructions towards the prevention and cure of chronic diseases peculiar to women; In which, their Nature is fully explained, and their Treatment, by Regimen and simple*

*Medicines, clearly laid down, divested of the Terms of Art, for the use of those affected with such Diseases, as well as the Medical Reader*. London: R. Baldwin, 1781.

Leiman, Jessica L. "'Booby's Fruitless Operations': The Crisis of Male Authority in Richardson's *Pamela*." *Eighteenth-Century Fiction* 22, no. 2 (2009–2010): 223–248.

Lennox, Charlotte. *The Female Quixote*. Oxford: Oxford University Press, 1989.

Lewis, Jeremy. Introduction to *Humphry Clinker*, by Tobias Smollett, vii–xxvii. London: Penguin Classics, 2008.

Lewis, Judith Schneid. *In the Family Way: Childbearing in the British Aristocracy, 1760–1860*. New Brunswick, NJ: Rutgers University Press, 1986.

Limon, John. *Stand-Up Comedy in Theory, or, Abjection in America*. Durham, NC: Duke University Press, 2000.

Lindemann, Mary. *Medicine and Society in Early Modern Europe*. New York: Cambridge University Press, 2010.

Lloyd, Josephine M. "The 'Languid Child' and the Eighteenth-Century Man-Midwife." *BHM* 75 (2001): 641–679.

Locke, John. *Essay Concerning Human Understanding*. 1689. Edited by Peter H. Nidditch. Oxford, UK: Clarendon, 1975.

———. *Two Treatises of Government*. 1689. Edited by Peter Laslett. New York: New American Library, 1965.

Lockwood, Thomas. "Fielding from Stage to Page." In *Henry Fielding: Novelist, Playwright, Journalist, Magistrate (1707–1754)*, edited by Claude Rawson, 21–39. Newark: Delaware University Press, 2008.

———. "Shamela." In *The Cambridge Companion to Henry Fielding*, edited by Claude Rawson, 39–49. Cambridge: Cambridge University Press, 2007.

———. "Theatrical Fielding." *Studies in the Literary Imagination* 32 (1999): 107–110.

Lord, Alexandra. "'The Great Arcana of the Deity': Menstruation and Menstrual Disorders in Eighteenth-Century British Medical Thought.' *Bulletin of the History of Medicine* 73 (1999): 38–63.

Loudon, Irvine. *Medical Care and the General Practitioner, 1750–1850*. Oxford, UK: Clarendon, 1986.

Lukács, Georg. *The Historical Novel*. Translated by Hannah Mitchell and Stanley Mitchell. London: Merlin, 1962.

Lund, Roger. "Laughing at Cripples: Ridicule, Deformity and the Argument from Design." *Eighteenth Century Studies* 39, no. 1 (2005): 91–114.

Lynch, James J. "Romance and Realism in Charlotte Lennox's *The Female Quixote*." *Essays in Literature* 14 (1987): 51–63.

Macafee, C.H.G. "The Obstetrical Aspects of *Tristram Shandy*." *Ulster Medical Journal* 19, no. 1 (1950): 12–22.

Mackenzie, James. *The History of Health*. Edinburgh: William Gordon, 1758.

Malina, Debra. "Rereading the Patriarchal Text: *The Female Quixote*, *Northanger Abbey*, and the Trace of the Absent Mother." *Eighteenth-Century Fiction* 8, no. 2 (1996): 271–292.

Manion, Jane. *Female Husbands: A Trans History*. Cambridge: Cambridge University Press, 2020.

Maubray, John. *The Female Physician*. London: James Holland, 1724.

Mauclerc, John Henry. *Dr. Blondel Confuted; or, The Ladies Vindicated, with Regard to the Power of Imagination in Pregnant Women: Together with a Circular and General Address to the Ladies, on This Occasion*. London: M. Cooper, 1747.

Mauriceau, François. *The Diseases of Women with Child and in Child-bed*. Translated by Hugh Chamberlen. London: John Darby, 1683.

McAllister, John. "Smollett's Semiology of Emotions: The Symptomology of the Passions and Affections in *Roderick Random* and *Peregrine Pickle*." *English Studies in Canada* 14 (1988): 286–295.

———. "Smollett's Use of Medical Theory: *Roderick Random* and *Peregrine Pickle*." *Mosaic* 22 (1989): 121–130.

McAllister, Marie E. "'Only to Sink Deeper': Venereal Disease in *Sense and Sensibility*." *Eighteenth-Century Fiction* 17, no. 1 (2004): 87–101.

McDonald, Michael. *Mystical Bedlam: Madness, Anxiety, and Healing in Seventeenth-Century England*. Cambridge: Cambridge University Press, 1981.

McKenzie, Alan T. *Certain Lively Episodes: The Articulation of Passion in Eighteenth-Century Prose*. Athens: University of Georgia Press, 1990.

McKeon, Michael. *The Origins of the English Novel, 1600–1740*. Baltimore: Johns Hopkins University Press, 2002.

———. *The Secret History of Domesticity: Public, Private, and the Division of Knowledge*. Baltimore: Johns Hopkins University Press, 2005.

McLaren, Angus. *Reproductive Rituals: The Perception of Fertility in England from the Sixteenth Century to the Nineteenth Century*. New York: Methuen, 1984.

McMaster, Juliet. "'Uncrystallized Flesh and Blood': The Body in *Tristram Shandy*." *Eighteenth-Century Fiction* 2, no. 3 (1990): 197–214.

———. "Walter Shandy, Sterne, and Gender: A Feminist Foray." In *Critical Essays on Laurence Sterne*, edited by Melvyn New, 198–214. New York: G. K. Hall, 1998.

McNamara, Tony. Screenplay for *Poor Things*. Directed by Yorgos Lanthimos. Searchlight Pictures, 2023.

Mead, Richard. *Medical Precepts and Cautions*. London: 1751.

Medoff, Jeslyn. "The Daughters of Behn and the Problem of Reputation." In *Women, Writing, History 1640–1740*, edited by Isobel Grundy and Susan Wiseman, 33–54. Athens: University of Georgia Press, 1992.

Meek, Heather. "'Meanders of [the] Purple Flood': Blood and Bloodletting in Eighteenth-Century Literature and Medicine." *Journal for Eighteenth-Century Studies* 46, no. 1 (2023): 41–57.

———. "Of Wandering Wombs and Wrongs of Women: Evolving Conceptions of Hysteria in the Age of Reason." *ECS* 35, nos. 2–3 (2009): 105–128.

Meigs, Charles D. *Woman: Her Diseases and Remedies*. Philadelphia: Blanchard and Lea, 1848.

Merchant, Carolyn. *The Death of Nature: Women, Ecology, and the Scientific Revolution*. San Francisco: Harper and Row, 1980.

Merians, Linda E., ed. *The Secret Malady: Venereal Disease in Eighteenth-Century Britain and France*. Lexington: University Press of Kentucky, 1996.

Michie, Allen. *Richardson and Fielding: The Dynamics of a Critical Rivalry*. Lewisburg, PA: Bucknell University Press, 1999.

Motooka, Wendy. *The Age of Reasons: Quixotism, Sentimentalism, and Political Economy in Eighteenth-Century Britain*. London: Routledge, 1998.

———. "Coming to a Bad End: Sentimentalism, Hermeneutics, and *The Female Quixote*." *Eighteenth-Century Fiction* 8 (1996): 251–270.

Mounsey, Chris. "Introduction: Variability: Beyond Sameness and Difference." In *The Idea of Disability in the Eighteenth Century*, edited by Chris Mounsey, 1–27. Lewisburg, PA: Bucknell University Press, 1997.

———. *Sight Correction: Vision and Blindness in Eighteenth-Century Britain*. Charlottesville: University of Virginia Press, 2019.

Müller, Johannes. *Elements of Physiology*. London: Taylor and Walton, 1839–1842.

Nance, Brian K. "Determining the Patient's Temperament: An Excursion into Seventeenth-Century Medical Semeiology." *Bulletin of the History of Medicine* 67, no. 3 (1993): 417–438.

Nicolazzo, Sal. "Henry Fielding's *The Female Husband* and the Sexuality of Vagrancy." *The Eighteenth Century* 55, no. 4 (2014): 335–353.

Nihell, Elizabeth. *A Treatise on the Art of Midwifery*. London: A. Morley, 1760.

Noggle, James. *Unfelt: The Language of Affect in the British Enlightenment*. Ithaca, NY: Cornell University Press, 2020.

Nussbaum, Felicity A. "'Savage' Mothers: Narratives of Maternity in the Mid-Eighteenth Century." *Cultural Critique*, no. 20 (1991): 123–151.

———. *Torrid Zones: Maternity, Sexuality, and Empire in Eighteenth-Century English Narratives*. Baltimore: Johns Hopkins University Press, 1995.

Paster, Gail Kern. *The Body Embarrassed: Drama and the Disciplines of Shame in Early Modern England*. Ithaca, NY: Cornell University Press, 1993.

Paulson, Ronald. *The Life of Henry Fielding: A Critical Biography*. Oxford, UK: Blackwell, 2000.

Paulson, Ronald, and Thomas Lockwood, eds. *Henry Fielding: The Critical Heritage*. London: Routledge, 1969.

Perry, Ruth. "Colonizing the Breast: Sexuality and Maternity in Eighteenth-Century England." *Journal of the History of Sexuality* 2, no. 2 (1991): 204–234.

———. *Novel Relations: The Transformation of Kinship in English Literature and Culture, 1748–1818*. Cambridge: Cambridge University Press, 2004.

———. "Words for Sex: The Verbal Sexual Continuum in *Tristram Shandy*." *Studies in the Novel* 20 (1988): 27–42.

Pilloud, Séverine, and Micheline Louis-Courvoisier. "The Intimate Experience of the Body in the Eighteenth Century: Between Interiority and Exteriority." *Medical History* 47, no. 4 (2003): 451–472.

Pollock, Linda. "Childbearing and Female Bonding in Early Modern England." *Social History* 22, no. 3 (1997): 286–306.

Pomata, Gianna. "Menstruating Men: Similarity and Difference of the Sexes in Early Modern Medicine." In *Generation and Degeneration: Tropes of Reproduction in Literature and History from Antiquity through Early Modern Europe*, edited by Valeria Finucci and Kevin Brownlee, 109–152. Durham, NC: Duke University Press, 2001.

Pope, Alexander. *An Epistle to a Lady*. 1735. In *Selected Poetry*, edited by Pat Rogers, 106–113. Oxford: Oxford University Press, 1998.

Porter, Roy. *English Society in the Eighteenth Century*. London: Penguin, 1991.

———. "'The Whole Secret of Health': Mind, Body and Medicine in *Tristram Shandy*." In *Nature Transfigured: Science and Literature, 1700–1900*, edited by John Christie and Sally Shuttleworth, 61–84. Manchester, UK: Manchester University Press, 1989.

Porter, Roy, and Dorothy Porter. *In Sickness and in Health: The British Experience 1650–1850*. London: Fourth Estate, 1988.

Potter, Tiffany. "'A Certain Sign That He Is One of Use': *Clarissa*'s Other Libertines." *Eighteenth-Century Fiction* 11, no. 4 (1999): 403–420.

———. *Honest Sins: Georgian Libertinism and the Plays and Novels of Henry Fielding*. Montreal: McGill-Queen's University Press, 1999.

Povey, Charles. *The Virgin in Eden; or, The State of Innocency*. London: J. Roberts, 1741.

*Present for Servants, A: From Their Ministers, Masters, or Other Friends*. 2nd ed. London: J. Downing, 1710.

Prytula, Nina. "'Great-Breasted and Fierce': Fielding's Amazonian Heroines." *Eighteenth Century Studies* 35, no. 2 (2002): 173–193.

Quétel, Claude. *History of Syphilis*. Translated by Judith Braddock and Brian Pike. Cambridge, UK: Polity, 1990.

Quillet, Claude. *La callipedie ou l'art d'avoir de beaux enfans*. Paris, 1749.

Raven, James. "From Promotion to Proscription: Arrangements for Reading and Eighteenth-Century Libraries." In *The Practice and Representation of Reading in England*, edited by James Raven, Helen Small, and Naomi Tadmor, 175–201. Cambridge: Cambridge University Press, 1996.

Richardson, Samuel. *Clarissa; or, The History of a Young Lady*. 1748. Reprint, London: Penguin, 1986.

———. *Pamela; or, With Virtue Rewarded*. 1740. Edited by T. C. Duncan Eaves and Ben D. Kimpel. Boston: Houghton Mifflin, 1971.

Richetti, John J. "Voice and Gender in Eighteenth-Century Fiction: Haywood to Burney." *Studies in the Novel* 19, no. 3 (1987): 263–272.

Richman, Jared S. "The Other King's Speech: Elocution and the Politics of Disability in Georgian Britain." *The Eighteenth Century* 59, no. 3 (2018): 279–304.

Risse, Guenter. "Hysteria at the Edinburgh Infirmary: The Construction and Treatment of a Disease, 1770–1800." *Medical History* 32, no. 1 (1988): 1–22.

Robbins, Bruce. *The Servant's Hand: English Fiction from Below*. New York: Columbia University Press, 1986.

Robinson, Nicholas. *A New System of the Spleen, Vapours, and Hypochondriack Melancholy*. London: Bettesworth, 1729.

Romanska, Magda, and Alan Ackerman. Introduction to *Reader in Comedy: An Anthology of Theory and Criticism*, edited by Magda Romanska and Alan Ackerman, 1–15. London: Bloomsbury, 2017.

Rosen, Aliza. "Important Abortion Cases in a Holding Pattern Following SCOTUS Decisions." Johns Hopkins: Bloomberg School of Public Health, July 3, 2024. https://publichealth.jhu.edu/2024/scotus-mifepristone-and-emtala-decisions-explained#:~:text=For%20now%2C%20mifepristone%20remains%20on,fire%20again%20in%20the%20future.

Ross, Deborah. "Mirror, Mirror: The Didactic Dilemma of *The Female Quixote*." *SEL* 27 (1987): 455–473.

Rousseau, G. S. "'Brainomania': Brain, Mind and Soul in the Long Eighteenth Century." *British Journal for Eighteenth-Century Studies* 30 (2007): 161–191.

———. "Matt Bramble and the Sulphur Controversy in the Eighteenth Century." *Journal of the History of Ideas* 28 (1967): 577–599.

———. "Pineapples, Pregnancy, Pica, and *Peregrine Pickle*." In *Tobias Smollett: Bicentennial Essays Presented to Lewis M. Knapp*, edited by G. S. Rousseau and P. G. Bouce, 79–110. New York: Oxford University Press, 1971.

Roussel, Pierre. *Système physique et moral de la femme, ou Tableau philosophique de la constitution, de l'état organique, du temperament, des moeurs, et des fonctions propres au sexe*. Paris, 1775.

Sawday, Jonathan. *The Body Emblazoned: Dissection and the Human Body in Renaissance Culture*. London: Routledge, 1996.

Schiebinger, Londa. *The Mind Has No Sex? Women in the Origins of Modern Science*. Cambridge, MA: Harvard University Press, 1989.

Scull, Andrew. *Hysteria: The Biography*. Oxford: Oxford University Press, 2009.

———. *The Most Solitary of Afflictions: Madness and Society in Britain, 1700–1900*. New Haven, CT: Yale University Press, 1993.

Scull, Andrew, and Diane Favreau. "The Clitoridectomy Craze." *Social Research* 53, no. 2 (1986): 243–260.

*Secret History of Pandora's Box*. London: T. Cooper, 1742.

Sedgwick, Eve Kosofsky. *Between Men: English Literature and Male Homosocial Desire*. New York: Columbia University Press, 1985.

Sermon, William. *The Ladies Companion; or, The English Midwife*. London: Edward Thomas, 1671.

Seth, Suman. *Difference and Disease: Medicine, Race, and the Eighteenth-Century British Empire*. Cambridge: Cambridge University Press, 2020.

Sheldon, Esther K. "What's an Impfiddle?" *American Speech* 50, nos. 1–2 (1975): 138–140.

Sheridan, Thomas. *Dissertation on the Causes of the Difficulties, Which Occur, in Learning of the English Tongue*. London: R. and J. Dodsley, 1762.

"Short Sermon on Matrimony, A." *Lady's Magazine*, October 1783.

Shorter, Edward. *From Paralysis to Fatigue: A History of Psychosomatic Illness in the Modern Era*. New York: Free Press, 1992.

Siena, Kevin. "'The Venereal Disease,' 1500–1800." In *The Routledge History of Sex and the Body, 1500 to the Present*, edited by Sarah Toulalan and Kate Fisher, 463–478. London: Routledge, 2013.

Sill, Geoffrey. "Robinson's Transgender Voyage: or, Burlesquing Crusoe." In *Robinson Crusoe after 300 Years*, edited by Andreas K. E. Mueller and Glynis Ridley, 27–60. Lewisburg, PA: Bucknell University Press, 2021.

Skinner, John. *Constructions of Smollett: A Study of Genre and Gender*. Newark: University of Delaware Press, 1996.

Smallwood, Angela J. *Fielding and the Woman Question*. New York: St. Martin's, 1989.

Smellie, William. *A Treatise on the Theory and Practice of Midwifery*. London: Alexander Cleugh and M. Watson, 1790.

Smith, Adam. *The Theory of Moral Sentiments*. 1759. Edited by Knud Haakonssen. Cambridge: Cambridge University Press, 2002.

Smollett, Tobias. *The Adventures of Ferdinand Count Fathom*. 1753. Edited by Jerry C. Beasley. Athens: University of Georgia Press, 2014.

———. *The Adventures of Peregrine Pickle*. 1751. Edited by James L. Clifford. Oxford: Oxford University Press, 1964.

———. *The Adventures of Roderick Random*. 1748. Edited by Paul-Gabriel Boucé. London: Oxford University Press, 1979.

———. *A Complete History of England, Deduced from the Descent of Julius Cæsar, to the Treaty of Aix la Chapelle, 1748. Containing the Transactions of One Thousand Eight Hundred and Three Years. By T. Smollett, M.D. . . .* Vol. 1. London: James Rivington and James Fletcher, 1757. Eighteenth Century Collections Online.

———. *The Expedition of Humphry Clinker*. 1771. Edited by James L. Thorson. New York: Norton, 1983.

Spacks, Patricia Meyer. "The Subtle Sophistry of Desire: Dr. Johnson and *The Female Quixote*." *Modern Philology* 85 (1988): 532–542.

*Spectator, The*. Vol. 5. London: Printed for S. Buckley and J. Tonson, 1713. Eighteenth Century Collections Online.

Spector, Robert D. *Smollett's Women: A Study in Eighteenth-Century Masculine Sensibility*. Westport, CT: Greenwood, 1994.

Spencer, Herbert R. *The History of British Midwifery: From 1650–1800*. New York: AMS Press, 1927.

Steele, Richard. *The Tatler*. Edited by Donald F. Bond. London: Oxford University Press, 1987.

Steele, Richard, and Joseph Addison. *The Spectator*. Edited by Donald F. Bond. London: Oxford University Press, 1965.

Sterne, Laurence. *The Life and Opinions of Tristram Shandy*. 1759. Edited by Ian Campbell Ross. Oxford: Oxford University Press, 2000.

Stolberg, Michael. "Self-Pollution, Moral Reform, and the Venereal Trade: Notes on the Sources and Historical Context of *Onania* (1716)." *Journal of the History of Sexuality* 9, no. 1 (2000): 37–61.

Strauss, Lévi. *The Elementary Structures of Kinship*. Boston: Beacon, 1969.

Strong-Cock, Paddy [pseud.]. *Teague-root Display'd: Being Some Useful and Important Discoveries Tending to Illustrate the Doctrine of Electricity*. London: W. Webb, 1746.

Studd, John. "A Comparison of 19th Century and Current Attitudes to Female Sexuality." *Gynecological Endocrinology* 23, no. 12 (2007): 673–681.

Stukeley, William. *Of the Spleen, Its Description and History*. London: Roberts, 1722.

Swift, Jonathan. *A Proposal for Correcting, Improving and Ascertaining the English Tongue*. London: Tooke, 1712.

Sydenham, Thomas. *Epistle to Dr. Cole*. In *The Works of Thomas Sydenham*, translated by R. D. Latham, 56–118. London: Sydenham Society, 1852.

Tadmor, Naomi. "The Concept of the Household-Family in Eighteenth-Century England." *Past and Present* 151 (1995): 111–140.

———. "'In the Even My Wife Read to Me': Women, Reading, and Household Life in the Eighteenth Century." In *The Practice and Representation of Reading in England*, edited by James Raven, Helen Small, and Naomi Tadmor, 162–174. Cambridge: Cambridge University Press, 1996.

Terry, Richard. "'P.S.': The Dangerous Logic of the Postscript in Eighteenth-Century Literature." *Modern Language Review* 109, no. 1 (2014): 35–53.

Thorson, James L. Preface to *The Expedition of Humphry Clinker*, by Tobias Smollett, xi–xv. New York: Norton, 1983.

Tierney-Hynes, Rebecca. *Novel Minds: Philosophers and Romance Readers, 1680–1740*. Basingstoke, UK: Palgrave Macmillan, 2012.

Tissot, Samuel. *De la santé des gens de lettres*. 1768. Introduction by Francois Azouvi. Geneva: Slatkine, 1981.

Todd, Janet. *The Sign of Angellica: Women, Writing and Fiction, 1660–1800*. New York: Columbia University Press, 1989.

Trotter, Thomas. *A View of the Nervous Temperament*. 3rd ed. Newcastle, UK: Walker, Longman, Hurst, Rees and Orme, 1812.

Tuana, Nancy. *The Less Noble Sex: Scientific, Religious and Philosophical Conceptions of Woman's Nature*. Bloomington: Indiana University Press, 1993.

Turner, Bryan. *The Body and Society: Explorations in Social Theory*. Thousand Oaks, CA: Sage, 1996.

Turner, Daniel. *De morbis cutaneis*. London: R. Bonwicke 1723.

Vogrinçic, Ana. "The Novel-Reading Panic in 18th-Century in England: An Outline of an Early Moral Media Panic." *Medijska istraživanja* 14, no. 2 (2008): 103–124.

Voltaire. *Philosophical Dictionary*. Translated by Theodore Besterman. Harmondsworth, UK: Penguin, 1971.

Wall, L. Lewis. "William Smellie (1697–1763), the Father of Scientific Obstetrics." *Medical Heritage* 2 (1986): 158–167.

Warren, Leland E. "Of the Conversation of Women: *The Female Quixote* and the Dream of Perfection." *Studies in Eighteenth-Century Culture* 11 (1982): 367–380.

Watson, Nicola. *Revolution and the Form of the British Novel, 1790–1825: Intercepted Letters, Interrupted Seductions*. Oxford, UK: Clarendon, 1994.

Wear, Andrew. *Knowledge and Practice in English Medicine 1550–1680*. Cambridge: Cambridge University Press, 2000.

Weed, David. "Sentimental Misogyny and Medicine in *Humphry Clinker*." *Studies in English Literature, 1500–1900*, 37, no. 3 (1997): 615–636.

"'Weep 'Weep!": History of Chimney Sweeps." *History Magazine* 12, no. 6 (2011): 42–44.

Wells, T. Spencer, Alfred Hegar, and Robert Battey. "Castration in Nervous Diseases: A Symposium." *American Journal of Medical Science* 92, no. 10 (1886): 455–490.

Whytt, Robert. *An Essay on the Vital and Involuntary Motions of Animals*. 1751. Reprint, Edinburgh: John Balfour, 1763.

———. *Observations on the Nature, Causes, and Cure of Those Disorders Which Are Commonly Called Nervous, Hypochondriac, or Hysteric. To Which Are Prefixed Some Remarks on the Sympathy of the Nerves, 1764*. London: T. Maiden, 1797.

———. *Physiological Essays*. Edinburgh: Hamilton, Balfour and Neill, 1761.

Wiehe, Jarred. "No Penis? No Problem: Intersections of Queerness and Disability in Laurence Sterne's *The Life and Opinions of Tristram Shandy, Gentleman*." *The Eighteenth Century* 58, no. 2 (2017): 177–193.

Wiesner-Hanks, Merry E. *Women and Gender in Early Modern Europe*. Cambridge: Cambridge University Press, 2000.

Wilson, Philip K., ed. *Childbirth: Changing Ideas and Practices in Britain and America 1600 to the Present*. New York: Garland, 1996.

Yeazell, Ruth. *Fictions of Modesty: Women and Courtship in the English Novel*. Chicago: University of Chicago Press, 1991.

Zach, Wolfgang. "Mrs Aubin and Richardson's Earliest Literary Manifesto (1739)." *English Studies* 62 (1981): 282–284.

Zaczek, Barbara Maria. *Censored Sentiments: Letters and Censorship in Epistolary Novels and Conduct Material.* Newark: University of Delaware Press, 1997.

Zigarovich, Jolene. "Transing the Gothic." In *TransGothic in Literature and Culture*, edited by Jolene Zigarovich, 1–22. London: Routledge, 2017.

# INDEX

## ABOUT THE AUTHOR

KATHLEEN TAMAYO ALVES is a professor of English at Queensborough Community College at The City University of New York. Her writings on eighteenth-century literature and culture, medicine, and literary history have appeared in *Studies in Eighteenth-Century Culture*, *Eighteenth-Century Fiction*, *Eighteenth-Century Studies*, and *The Eighteenth Century: Theory and Interpretation*.